FIRST FUN

Sheila Gregory and Diane Melvin

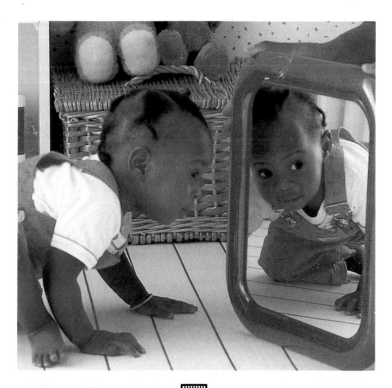

Villard Books **V** New York 1986

CONTENTS

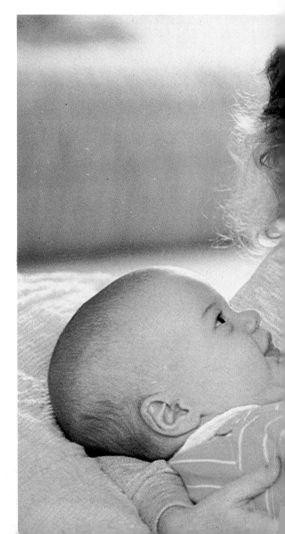

All rights reserved under International and Pan-American Copyright Conventions. Published in the United States by Villard Books, a division of Random House, Inc., New York, and simultaneously in Canada by Random House of Canada Limited, Toronto. First published in Great Britain by Conran Octopus Limited in 1984.

Library of Congress Catalog Card Number: 84-40576
ISBN: 0-394-54476-5

Printed and bound in Hong Kong
9 8 7 6 5 4 3 2
First American Edition

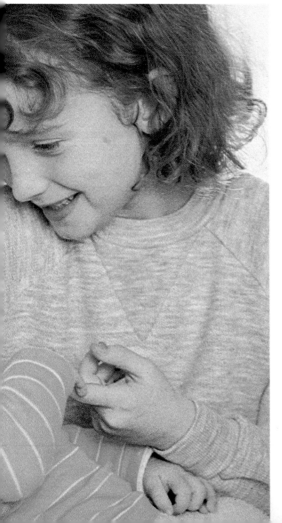

INTRODUCTION

During the first two years of life your baby grows into a child. He develops from a helpless newborn into a capable toddler who looks very like a little adult. You can have lots of fun watching him grow, joining in his play and sharing with him the new things that every day offers.

You will be thrilled by his first steps and words. These are the milestones you remember in the future. But the little changes, each building on the one before, are just as important though easily overlooked.

The chapters in this book follow your baby's progress and the different ways he plays during his first two years. There are lots of ideas for games to play with him and toys he'll like. We hope these ideas will help you enjoy your developing baby and have fun together.

Let's have fun

All the toys and playthings described in this book have proved very popular with babies and young children as well as helping them to play and learn. Many of the toys can be used in different ways by babies of different ages. You will find as your baby grows older that he returns to his favorite toys and includes them in new games.

Play is essential to your baby's progress. When he is sitting on your lap he may touch your clothes and then reach for a toy, showing you that he wants to play and will use everything he can as a toy. He learns through play, but he needs some help to get the most out of it. There will be times when he may not feel like playing because he's tired or unwell. This won't last long and soon he'll be back to his usual self, eagerly finding new playthings to fill his day.

There are some things that all babies need in order to develop and show you what they are able to do. One of the most important things is the security you provide, by showing him that you're interested in what he's doing. By thinking about what toys will please him and watching his changing needs, you are giving him the opportunity to try out new skills. Your companionship is precious to him, but as he grows he will also enjoy playing with other adults and friends too. A mother-and-toddler group gives him new toys to play with in new surroundings. A balance between old and new, between enjoying individual attention and joining in a group, is the situation in which he can best play, develop and thrive. He needs both security and challenges to help him progress.

Being a mother is a time of many changes; sometimes you may wonder if you'll ever get it right. You will get it right because you *can* provide the things he needs in these early years. If relatives and friends always seem to be comparing what your baby can do with what another one is doing, remember that babies, like adults, are all different. Your baby may crawl at an early stage but talk at a late one; or he may be able to say many more words than a friend the same age, while not building a tower of blocks as well. Although there are these differences, all babies follow the

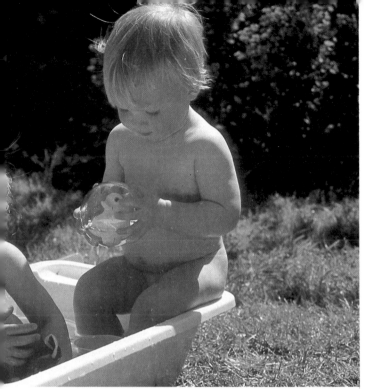

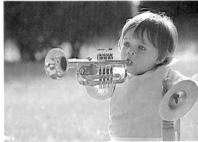

him; he can copy your actions; he can move his arms and wrist, and he can recognize the friend to wave to. These are just four of the many skills involved in a seemingly simple action. Small steps forward like these lead to large ones and watching them happen as you play with your child and his toys is part of the fun.

There are a small number of toys which your baby or toddler will probably enjoy at any time:

Blocks
Action toys
Ball
You

Picture book
Large toy
A noise-making toy
Your things
Soft toys

When you're looking for toys, remember BABY PLAYS and it will remind you of some of the basic playthings.

same basic pattern of progress — they learn to sit before they move or walk; they babble before they talk.

All babies are different, and so are their mothers. Each baby has likes and dislikes, and you too are entitled to tolerate some things while others drive you frantic! Life for each baby is different and this will influence the way he views the world.

The more closely you watch your child develop, the more you will enjoy the small changes as well as the large ones. As you hear his first words you'll think back to his first "noises." Those early sounds lead to babbles; then he uses certain babbles in particular situations. Slowly these sound more and more like parts of words. When he shows you something new, such as waving "bye-bye," he is showing you in one action that he has progressed in many ways. Now he can understand what you're saying to

Baby can

Your newborn baby can see and hear you and will soon be smiling and reaching for his first toys.

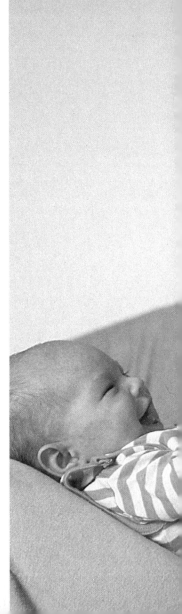

As soon as your baby is born he has so much to learn, both about you and about the world into which he has been born. The early stages in his development are as important as any of his future achievements: they form the foundations on which all later progress is built. You will get to know much more about him as he develops.

In these early days you may wonder what your baby will be like as he grows, and whether you are doing the right things to help him get the most out of what the world has to offer. If you can simply be with him, giving him all the attention you can, receiving all the pleasure he can give you, you will be helping him. The time you spend together in these early days is what most helps his progress.

In the early weeks he will be learning to make some sense of what he hears, sees and feels.

A new baby's skills
(0-8 weeks)
It's easy to underestimate what a helpless-looking newborn baby can do; but watch him – he can do lots of things. Almost every day you will notice some changes in what he can do. Even though these changes may be small and only noticeable to you, they are

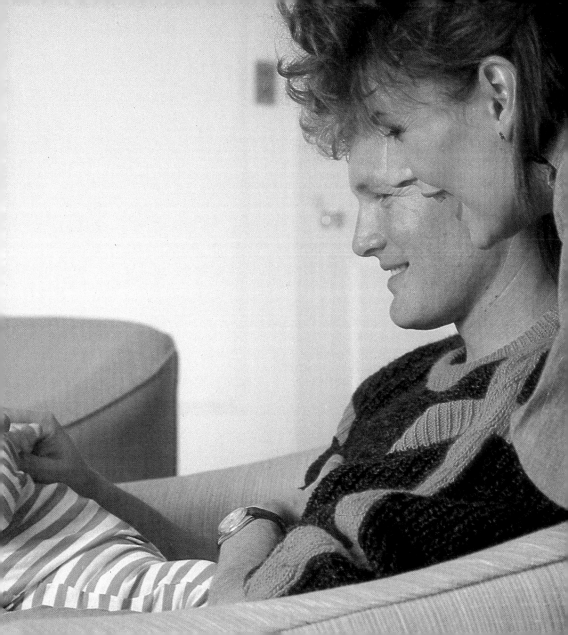

very important. Later progress could not happen without them. For example, your baby would not be able to sit up without first being able to hold his head up and keep his back straight.

Essential skills

Some of your baby's early skills are necessary for his survival.

Crying. He can ask you to provide what he needs by crying, his main way of getting your attention. Before long you'll be able to pick up different cries, for when he's hungry, tired, in pain, or just bored!

Sucking. He also needs to be able to suck and swallow so he can take in his feedings. Sucking is an action he is capable of even before birth, as photographs of babies in the womb sucking their fingers have shown. While he cannot find his own way to the breast or bottle, the smell and sight of food will make him move his mouth and tongue in anticipation (this is called rooting). Soon he'll learn to turn his head slightly so that his mouth comes into contact with the nipple or bottle nipple. Stroking his cheek lightly on the side nearest the milk may encourage him to turn his head.

Physical contact

The pleasure he gets from being held close to you can be seen right from birth too. His body seems to mold into yours when you hold him close; watch how he snuggles down when you cuddle him in your arms. He might like being in a baby sling or carrier. Choose one which holds him close to your body while supporting his head and back. Crying and sucking are obviously necessary for him to survive, but this early contact with you is no less important. It gives him a sense of security and protection which he must have to progress and it deepens the feelings that make you and your baby special to each other. His awareness of well-being and comfort becomes linked to all the people who care for him.

The baby's senses

Seeing. At birth your baby's senses are ready to cope with all the new sights, sounds, textures and smells he will experience. A newborn baby's eyes will follow a slowly moving object which is held close to him. Striking or colorful patterns attract him, and so does the human face he especially likes to look at – yours. He may look up and "search" your face and eyes when cradled in your arms. In this position your face is probably at the best distance – 8-10 inches (20-25 cm) from his own – for him to focus clearly on it. Very soon he will begin to reach up and explore it with his hands.

Hearing. Your newborn baby can hear and, although he does not know what different noises mean, he shows a liking for certain kinds of sounds. Rhythmical sounds, especially your voice talking or singing gently, may soothe your baby if he's restless. He may quiet a little as you talk when approaching him in his crib or if you play a music box to him. Gradually, as he gains more control over his movements, he will start to turn his eyes and then later his head towards the place where the sound is coming from. In these early days a sudden noise may startle him if he is waking up. Yet if he's deeply asleep a loud noise won't disturb him.

Reflexes

Although a newborn baby cannot support his own head, and has very little control over how his limbs move, he does have a number of spontaneous movements. These are reflexes which are present at birth but gradually disappear. One reflex which you can trigger is the grasp reflex. If you stroke the palm of his hand with your finger, his fingers will close firmly around yours. This is not the same as the deliberate

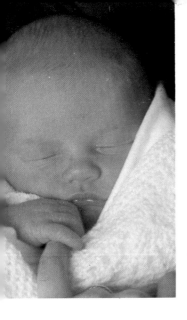

Your newborn baby can grip your fingers surprisingly strongly; this is one of his early reflexes.

action he will make later on when holding toys.

Early development

If your baby is happy to lie in different positions for short times this will help strengthen his muscles. Lying on his tummy, for example, will encourage him to lift his head up and strengthen his back and neck. On his back, he will be able to see more and may start turning his head to follow moving objects. At this early stage you may find that he will quickly get restless or upset if left for long in a new position.

It is remarkable how quickly your baby shows changes in what he can do. When you're holding him you will probably feel him straighten his head a little, kick his legs and move his arms. These are some of the skills the doctor will look for at the first developmental check-up when your baby is about one month old. The doctor may look at your baby's head control and his posture both lying flat and when pulled to sitting as well as checking on which reflexes are still present. At this age your baby is too young for a complete assessment of hearing or eyesight. Nevertheless the doctor will ask you if your baby can hear and may check the beginnings of listening by the way he reacts to noises. The baby at this age hasn't usually started to smile but stares intently at your face.

First smiles

Sometimes even very tiny babies offer smiles, but they are fleeting and it's not always clear what caused them. By two months, however, most babies will look up at you and then a smile will very deliberately spread across their faces. Your baby may smile readily at anyone at this time, but soon his smiles will be reserved for his special friends.

Your baby has now learned a lot

about the world but he still has a long way to go. You'll have learned about him too, finding out what he likes and what upsets him. His personality is beginning to show itself: he may be a noisy or restless baby or a quiet and placid one. He might sleep for long periods or prefer a lot of short naps. These preferences point to the kind of child he may become but his daily behavior is mainly a result of how hungry, tired or uncomfortable he is.

The new baby's day

Much of your baby's time in the early weeks is taken up with feeding and sleeping. If he takes a long time to nurse or is difficult to settle afterwards, it can seem as if your whole day is taken up keeping him content, leaving little time for anything else. It may help both you and your baby to introduce some routines into the day, setting a pattern which will continue as he grows.

At first you may find it is your baby who sets the overall pace and pattern of the day. On some days he may be particularly wakeful or unsettled, on others hungry or sleepy; it can be difficult to plan ahead. Too many visits or arrangements in one day can be exhausting for both of you in the first weeks. However, trying to

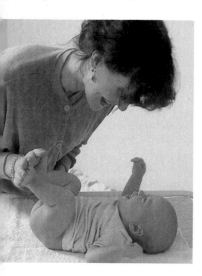

Changing time, and bath time too, are opportunities to play with your baby; he'll love it if you pedal his feet.

Toys for the new baby

Your newborn baby's best toy is you. He'll enjoy being carried by you, looking up at your face, hearing your voice talking or singing to him. It's through you that he learns about other objects as you show him what's going on around him and talk to him.

Mobiles and moving toys

There are some toys to buy or make which your baby will like, and which will be useful later. He'll be attracted by gently moving objects, for example: chime bars, mobiles, toy windmills and cradle play toys all encourage him to look and follow the movement. A musical mobile may be especially successful in getting his interest. Don't hang it high up from the ceiling because it will be too far away for him to see while lying in his crib; hang it low or hold him up near to it.

Making a crib play toy. It's easy to make a crib play toy yourself. Fix a piece of cord (not elastic) or a bar securely across the crib and suspend a variety of things from it, such as shiny colored paper discs, a little key or two, a ball with a bell inside, a small teddy bear or empty spools tied together. Make sure all the objects are firmly tied on and the cord is securely fixed at each end. Don't choose anything which

get out each day, even for a short walk, can give you both a welcome break.

At changing time give him the chance to kick without the restrictions of a diaper. His legs very soon begin to make more definite movements and he may push against your hands when you hold them against his feet. Bathtime is another opportunity for kicking – some babies love the feeling of the water around them and they will kick and splash.

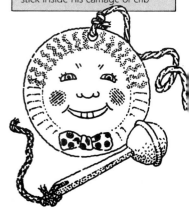

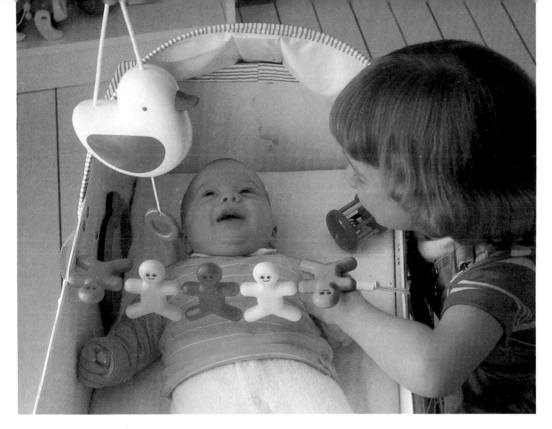

A very young baby will love bright toys that move and make a noise.

might be dangerous or could be swallowed if it did come off, like little beads or long strings. The advantage of home-made mobiles is that you can change the objects from time to time.

Carriage toys

To give your baby something to look at when he's awake, string big bright beads across his carriage or stroller or hang a brightly colored rattle or a paper plate with the outline of a face drawn on it in front of him. At this age your baby can focus on objects best if they are 8-12 inches (20-30 cm) away from him. Colored pictures, especially with reds or greens, or bright patterns placed on the side of his crib or carriage are close enough for him

to see if he lies on his side. The movements in a baby mirror may also attract him.

Listening toys

The soft tune of a musical box can help soothe your baby if he is upset or restless. If you play it when you settle him for his night sleep it will help him to realize it's time for bed.

Collect or make a few rattles that feel and sound different.

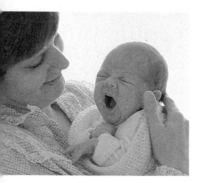

The day can prove quite tiring for a very young baby!

Games to play

Even in these very early weeks there may be times when your baby is happy to be awake. Hold him close in front of you with your hands cupped around the back of his head and his back resting against your arms so that he can look straight at you. He'll love being rocked gently back and forth. Now you can talk to him quietly; see how his eyes gaze intently at you. It won't be long before he starts to join in with your "conversation" – taking turns with you by slightly nodding his head, moving his eyes and mouth, "smiling" or "grimacing." Later on he'll join in with gurgles and laughs. Hearing your voice is a crucial part of his learning about talking.

Skills of the infant
(2-6 months)

As the weeks pass your new baby will be progressing quickly. The muscles on his neck and back grow stronger. He'll move his head and eyes in an effort to see as much as possible. He can now fix his gaze on something of interest and follow its movement.

Looking and learning

When lying on his back, he can look upwards for quite a time, holding his head still without it flopping over to the side. Mobiles come into their own now and he'll start to notice things when he's out in the carriage. The movements of trees in the wind may particularly fascinate him. He'll also like to watch his own movements, not knowing that he is making them. At first you may see him looking at one of his outstretched hands for a moment. As he gently turns it, opens and shuts it, he becomes more absorbed. At about four months old he may start bringing both hands into play together and begin to touch his fingers.

You can make playtime more interesting for him by propping him up for short periods so that he can look around, free to turn his head and use his arms. Remember that his head and back need support and that he may tire quickly. Don't leave him alone. A bouncing chair or a low reclining baby chair is useful, and can be carried from room to room.

Keeping busy. As your baby is probably awake for longer now he'll need something to occupy him to prevent him from getting bored or restless. Watching you doing everyday household jobs – washing up, ironing, weeding the garden – offers him a whole range of new sounds and sights, and being near whoever is looking after him adds to his contentment. Chatting to him while you work will help him feel involved, and forms an important step in building a language of his own.

Watching other children will also fascinate him at this age. Toddlers may be a bit too boisterous for him to cope with at times, and they may not be tolerant of tiny babies. You will have to keep an eye on what's going on; but older children can be very good at including a baby in their play, talking to him or calling out his name now and again.

Joining in

It won't be long before your baby starts to join in whatever he's watching, waving his arms in excitement, laughing and gurgling or making sounds of his own. Shouts, exclamations and the sounds that are simplest to make such as "coo" and "gaa" come first. You'll notice that he enjoys repeating these sounds, delighting in his achievement, and now tries to copy the noises you make. When, at around three or four months, he can turn his head to find out where different noises are coming from, feedings may be interrupted. He may decide to stop sucking to discover who's talking, what made that noise at the door, and so on. He wants to be involved in everything!

While listening and making his own sounds are important at this age, it's what he *sees* that has the greatest impact. For example, his first smiles were brought out by the combination of your voice and your face. Gradually your voice alone becomes less likely to make him smile but your face, and later just a picture of your face, will continue to make him beam with excitement.

Reaching and grasping

The scene is now set for him to move on from watching to reaching and grasping. Reaching involves many skills, all of which must come together for your baby to do it effectively: his muscles need to be strong enough to support and turn his head; he must be able to focus on objects further away as well as notice the

small details, and he needs to have some control over his arm to keep it steady and guide his hand towards the right place as he reaches out. Watching all these skills come together, seeing how step by step he gets better at reaching, is great fun.

A bold wave of the arm in the vague direction of a suspended toy may be the first step. He may accidentally touch it, then take a more purposeful swipe. In time, he'll guide his arm to the toy and close his hand around it. He learns to grasp or hold objects in the same way, one step at a time. At first, he can briefly hold on to an object you place in his hand, but he doesn't seem to know it's there and it soon drops without his noticing it. Soon he starts to look at the toy and move it so he can see it better. When he can reach out and grab it, he'll put it to his mouth, shake it or bang it. Quite soon he begins holding small toys or rattles in both hands, but will not pass the toy from one hand to another until he is older.

Cuddles and contact

Although sometimes content to sit and watch, he is still very much in need of contact with you, and it's nice for you both to have a quiet cuddle. Don't worry, you won't spoil him by spending some of your spare minutes just

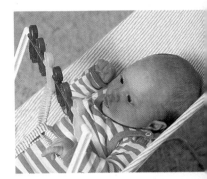

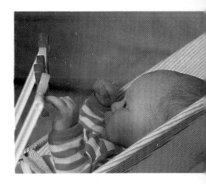

It's fun to see how your baby's first quite accidental, swipes (top) soon become deliberate movements as he learns to reach out and grasp things.

enjoying his company. Even if you are a working mother there will be some time to share with him. It is not necessarily the length of time you are together but what you do in that time that is important for your baby.

BABY CAN (birth to 6 months)

	watching ➡	reaching ➡	holding ➡
Making sense of the world	He is aware of changes in his surroundings but is not able to produce changes himself	Beginning to reach and cause effects in his surroundings Interacting with people	➡
Whole body control	Holds his head still for only a moment He enjoys lying in a position where he gets total support for his body – on his back, side or tummy	Lifts his head up for a while while lying on his tummy He can sit propped up for a while if his head and back are supported	➡
Looking	He looks at a brightly colored object held near him and may follow briefly with his eyes if it moves He "peers" up at an adult's face and watches their eyes and mouth move	Turns his head to follow a moving object and watches for longer He watches his own fingers and hands move	➡
Using his hands	Tends to hold his hands with his fingers closed Waves arms and hands about but not in any direction	He holds on to things briefly if they are placed in his hand He reaches out towards an object to touch it	➡
Listening	Sudden loud noises startle him when he is awake A quiet voice soothes him (especially if he is held and rocked too)	New sounds catch his interest and he searches for them with his eyes Beginning to repeat his own noises – "coos" and "gaa's," etc.	➡
Communicating	Cries and wriggles to show he needs something He may show some brief smiles	He makes a variety of sounds and movements in play Smiles and laughs at people	➡
Looking after himself	Relies on others to do things for him but he can turn to *suck* and swallow his milk and can *cry* for attention	Starting to hold on to his bottle when feeding Appeals to adults to pick him up and play by stretching and gurgling	➡

The infant's day

During the first two or three months you and your baby learn quite a lot about each other. You can often tell when he's tired and ready for a nap, even if his need for sleep varies from day to day. Certainly different babies need different amounts of sleep. Gradually you'll learn the best way to settle him down: which position he finds comfortable, whether he likes to be tightly wrapped up, or to be rocked for a while. He may like a pacifier or his fingers to suck.

Starting a routine

You may want to start establishing a routine for bedtime. Try putting your baby in different clothes; lay him in a different place or room from where he takes naps in the day; have a quiet wash-and-change time, maybe singing softly to him or playing musical toys. You'll soon find your own ways of showing him that it's bedtime.

Try to be flexible when organizing your day, as routines often have to be varied according to your baby's mood. *Your* mood will also determine how to cope. Sometimes you can drop everything and attend to him; at others he has to wait. If your baby has regular sleeping times, it is easier to plan the day.

Your more wakeful baby

In the course of the early weeks your baby will probably start to spend less and less time asleep. At first much of his waking time was taken up by feedings. Even then he may only have been fully awake for a few minutes or so then dozed off for a short nap in the middle. As he grows he can stay awake for longer in the day. During these times he will really enjoy your company and will benefit most from some variety in what he does. Move him around from place to place. Try laying him on his back or tummy on a changing mat or on the floor, to give him different views of the world and give him the chance to practice looking around and lifting his head up.

All babies cry from time to time and yours may be cranky at certain times of the day. A soothing bath or bottle, carrying him round in a sling, shaking a rattle, are all possible means of soothing a crying baby. However, there will be times when everything you've tried to distract or settle him has failed and you will need to take a deep breath and control your feelings of frustration.

Being a parent

Both mother and father have an important part to play and the more time the father can spend

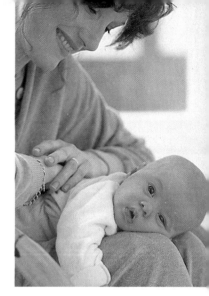

Your baby will enjoy close contact which makes him feel secure.

with his baby, the sooner he will learn to know him. Perhaps helping to settle him in the evening, or taking him out in his carriage at weekends, could be times for father to spend with baby – and let you have a little free time.

Your baby's need for entertainment will take up an increasing amount of your time. Most mothers have days when they wonder if their lives will ever return to normal. You might want to join a local mother-and-baby group, where you will find that many of your feelings are shared by other mothers.

Toys and playthings

Throughout his early life, you and any others who look after him are your baby's most important playthings. People give him something to watch, listen to and touch and through you he gets to know about other objects and toys.

Toys to look at

The most interesting toys for him now are those that are stimulating to look at: as well as mobiles, a bouncy toy on a loose spring or colorful rattle suspended on a piece of cord will encourage him first to take swipes, then reach out and touch it. He is becoming more co-ordinated.

To keep his interest, switch one item on his crib toy at a time. If you use small lengths of fine elastic to attach the objects on the mobile, this will produce an interesting effect as a light touch or kick by your baby will cause the objects to bounce up and down.

A colorful merry-go-round which moves freely on a pivot or a carousel which plays a gentle tune can help him learn to concentrate for longer periods. Chime bells, which move easily when touched or kicked and produce interesting sounds, may also fascinate him and encourage him to move his arms and legs. A pop-up doll makes a "peek-a-boo"

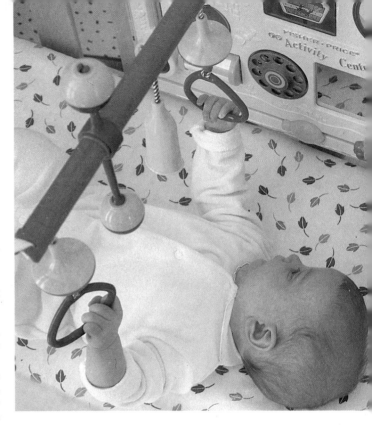

Your older baby will enjoy toys that he can reach out and touch.

game more fun, and the surprise is not so sudden or startling that it frightens him.

Toys to touch

An activity center or board is a good buy. It gives him plenty to look at if put in the side of his crib or hung on a playpen. As it will encourage him to reach out, the board should include at least one part which moves easily. Since his hands are not yet capable of pressing or turning things some of the parts have a use later on, so this purchase will have a long life.

Give your baby different objects to grapple with to encourage him to become more skillful with his hands. Choose things that are non-breakable, non-toxic, with no sharp edges and too

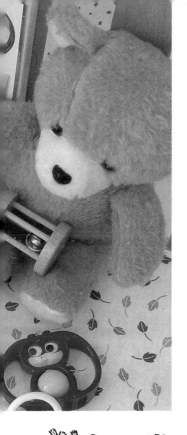

Toys to buy

1. Mobiles with a variety of colorful attachments
2. Fascinating toys – merry-go-rounds and carousels; chime balls or transparent balls with a spinning device inside; pop-up dolls
3. Rattles, shakers and teethers made of both wood and plastic to give variety
4. Activity center with parts requiring only a simple action
5. Soft toy – small teddy bear, rag doll, etc.
6. Simple board picture books

Toys to make

1. Rummage box – collect a boxful of safe everyday objects of different textures for handling or for suspending on cord to make your own mobile. Examples include painted spools, clothes-pins, pieces of cloth
2. Pop-up doll made from a dish mop with ribbons, bells, or paper face attached. Poke this through a used detergent bottle, cut in half

large to swallow. As they are soon likely to go into his mouth, it helps if they are washable too. As well as safe household objects which he can hold (clothespins, spoons, and so on) a rattle will probably be one of the first toys he handles. When you choose a rattle, look for one with a part which will fit into his tiny hand – the teething or keyring type or ones just shaped like "dumb-bells" are most suitable. Rattles should give variety in the noise they make as well as the way they feel. Wooden rattles feel and sound different from plastic ones. Later on he will be using his fingers as well as his whole hand to explore.

Other kinds of useful early toys include small teddy bears, rag dolls or soft animals that have limbs or ears which can be grasped easily by a tiny hand. A ball with knobs or indentations in it for holding is another good buy.

First books

Board or plastic books, especially those with big pictures of every-day objects, are useful in a baby's first years. Even at this stage he will probably enjoy watching you turn the pages and talk as he sits on your lap. As he grows older he will begin to point at the objects that become familiar.

Games to play

In quiet moments when you are talking to your baby and playing with him he will be joining in more and more, gaining ever greater pleasure from your company. He may try to copy you, blinking deliberately, blowing bubbles or even making some noises as if he were trying to talk back to you. His hands may start moving too. Ask him questions when you talk to him and he'll want to join in even more. The change in your tone of voice will interest him; your eyes opening wider and eyebrows going up – all these will make him watch you. If he starts to lose interest in these "conversations" bring a toy near and include it in your talk to revive his attention. Although he doesn't know the meaning of your words, he seems to listen very intently.

Watching and listening

He's most attentive when sitting propped up and fully awake. He'll soon be able to follow a small colored toy if you move it slowly in front of him, from one side to the other and up and down. Once he can do this easily, make the toy disappear behind a piece of paper or cardboard. Ask him: "Where's it gone?" Then make it re-emerge the other side: "There it is!" At first he will probably have

no idea where to look once it has disappeared. In a few weeks he will begin to look towards the spot where it will reappear.

He may also enjoy simple listening games when sitting up. Ring a toy bell or rattle out of his eyesight and at about 12-14 inches (30-35 cm) away from one ear.

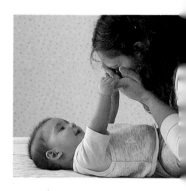

Your baby will love touching you and playing an early game of peek-a-boo.

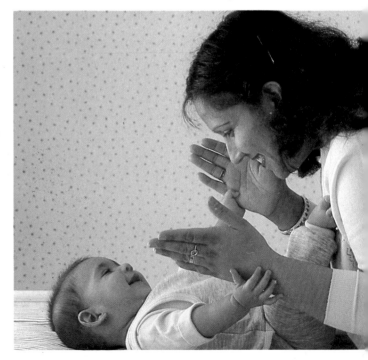

At first he may look for a sound. Soon he'll turn his head to find it.

Physical games

He'll have a great time playing games that involve touching you – pulling your hair, poking your face or mouth, or tugging at your clothes, and he'll like it when you touch him back, giving him little tickles to make him laugh or gurgle. You'll find yourself using your own nonsense words or singing made-up rhymes.

Your baby is probably more active now, kicking his legs and waving his arms with great gusto. He'll make these actions repeatedly, especially if they cause interesting things to happen like making the objects on a mobile move or causing great splashes in the bath. Patting his tummy, pedaling his feet and bouncing him gently on your knee will prepare him for more energetic games, if he seems to like them. Some babies enjoy being taken swimming at this age too. You will know how much he can tolerate at any one time. Some days he will not want to be bounced around at all, while on others he'll want more boisterous activities to go on and on.

Remember that a young baby can get bored and likes plenty of variety because he can't concentrate for very long on anything.

Safety

How can you ensure that your baby experiences different things in a safe way?

- It is baby's personal safety which is important at this age, as he has very little contact with objects. He needs support for his head and back, especially when being picked up and moved around.
- Since your baby can do little for himself, he is very vulnerable. He depends on you to think ahead and plan a safe environment for him; at bathtime, for example, you should make sure the water is not too hot. Never, never leave him alone in the bath, not even for a moment. Do not lay him down on a pillow in his carriage or crib. Do not use any toys on strings that could wind round his neck or anything in which his fingers could become entangled. Dispose of plastic bags – on new clothes, toys and so on – the minute you unwrap them.
- When he starts to handle and hold toys, consider carefully what you give him. For example, if you use elastic or cord for a toy, take care that any one piece is not too long – he won't understand the danger of wrapping it around himself.

Even the very best toys can become dangerous in the wrong hands. A good toy for a three year old could be lethal to a baby who is putting everything in his mouth.

Don't assume that all toys sold in stores are safe. You must judge for yourself whether a toy is appropriate for your baby or toddler. Be careful to avoid:

sharp objects and edges
small detachable parts which could be put in the mouth
poisonous paint
toys which are not easily cleaned
stuffed animals with glass or button eyes that could be pulled off
flammable toys
internal wires that could protrude with wear

Remember also to remove decorative bows before giving soft toys to a young baby – he could put the ribbon into his mouth and choke.

Now I can sit

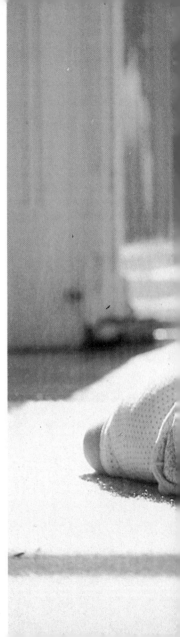

Once your baby can sit he'll be able to reach out for his own toys and will be babbling away to himself as he plays.

When you see your baby sitting alone for the first time, you'll realize the tremendous strides he has made in the first few months of his life. Sitting brings a greater degree of independence. As his hands are free, he can play in quite a different way, and he has acquired many other new skills as well. He enjoys looking for toys, reaching for them, picking them up and feeling them with his mouth. He may have started to babble and, to your delight, may say "dadadada" or "mama." These are not his first words, however, but experiments with sounds. All the time he is showing you how he is building on the things he has learned in the months before. Having learned to look, reach, hold and sit, he can put these together and hold a cup. He can direct his hands and bang a toy or play with his food. He is taking an active part in family life.

This growing independence is exciting, but also makes more demands on you – and you have many other demands to fulfill, especially if you have an older child. Start looking on your own activities as games to play rather than duties to perform and you'll see that some everyday chores, like emptying grocery bags for example, can be transformed into playtimes.

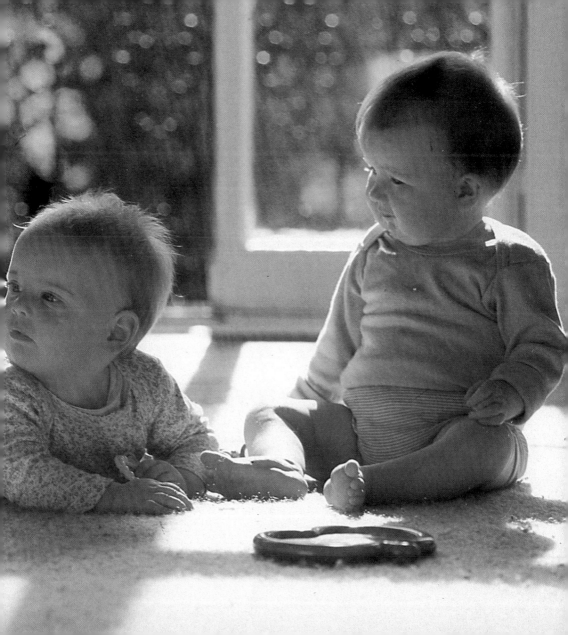

Skills of the baby who can sit

Your baby's ability to control his own movements, as in all things, develops gradually.

Learning to sit

At first, your baby can only sit alone for a few seconds before flopping to one side. Put some cushions on either side of him to give him extra support. Now he can see the world in quite a different way from when he was lying down. When making his first attempts to sit, all his effort is taken up in trying to balance. He cannot yet hold a toy at the same time or reach for a new one. Until he can do so – and it won't be long – put his toys on a tray clipped on to his chair, or string them across his bouncing chair or stroller.

Sitting and reaching

Gradually your baby will sit more steadily, and will be able to sit for longer periods. He can balance, reach forward and maybe turn around. Since he no longer fears flopping to one side, he can use his arms and hands for play rather than to balance. Some babies reach this stage very quickly and are sitting steadily by seven to eight months. Others, quite normally, take their time.

Beginning to roll

Even babies who can sit up will still spend time playing on their tummies or backs. They also like to feel the ground under their feet when you hold them up in a standing position. When your baby is on his tummy he may try to roll. At first it is easier for him to roll from his back on to his stomach. Now he will need more space; a large playmat will protect him from hard surfaces. If his toys are within easy reach he may roll purposefully to get them.

Using his hands

The way in which your baby uses his hands is also changing. When he picks up a toy, he cups his whole hand around it. He likes to grasp the handle of a rattle or spoon, or a small block. Gradually he is gaining more control of his arms. He can knock toys down, wave, pull a toy on a string towards him, pass a toy from one hand to another, crumple paper and play with two toys at once. As he learns to use his fingers and thumb in different ways, he'll be able to pick up smaller and more complex objects. By the time he is eight to twelve months old he has what is known as a pincer grip, when he picks up small objects using his thumb and first finger. This new skill brings potentially dangerous objects within his grasp, like bits of soft tissue, cookies or beads which

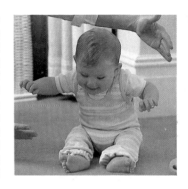

Though very wobbly at first (above) your baby will soon be sitting steadily (right) and reaching for toys. Now he can pick up small objects just using his finger and thumb (far right).

he'll stuff in his mouth, up his nose or in his ears given half a chance. Don't leave things like this lying around, and keep a constant eye on your baby.

Skill with his hands means that your baby can now do more for himself, holding his own cup or bottle, pulling at his clothes. These little changes are very important to his independence and his confidence in what he can do. But he still needs you, and will reach up to you when he wants to be picked up and given a big hug. He's showing his emotions more – he laughs at himself in a mirror, and will get upset if a toy is taken away from him.

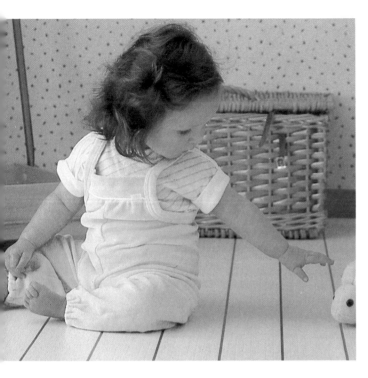

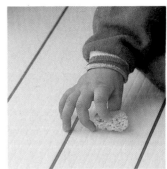

back to him, laughing at him or repeating his own sounds, he'll be encouraged to try again or gurgle and laugh at you. He is beginning to make an important link between objects (his toys) and sounds. A fascinating toy such as a music box may catch his eye and he will react noisily to draw your attention to it as well.

Starting to move
It's towards the end of this stage that some babies make their first attempts to move around, by pulling themselves up on a chair or a nearby leg! Maybe there's a special toy he's trying to reach. He may roll right across his play-mat on to the floor or turn around on his tummy. He may even try to crawl. At first he may go back-wards and seem confused and delighted at the same time by the outcome of his efforts. You may have been waiting and watching

Babbling
All the time, your baby is trying hard to communicate with you. He has more control over his maturing vocal cords, and he can make a wide range of sounds and repeat new ones which he hears. He's learning to listen. When you want to show him a book or play with his toys, make sure you have his attention first. This is especially important if he is

frequently blocked up with a cold and finds it more difficult to hear.

The first sounds your baby makes are what are called "single syllable sounds," like "ba ba" and "ga ga." Later on he will join these two sounds together and say "ba ba ga ga" or " dada mama." Some-times he will look at you or your friends and hold a long conversa-tion, chatting in a language he alone understands. If you talk

NOW I CAN SIT (around 6 to 9 months)

	sitting ⇒	holding and doing ⇒	moving ⇒
Making sense of the world	Exploring objects and his toys by reaching, mouthing, banging and grabbing One object is easily replaced by another	He explores his toys more purposefully (2 objects banged together, shaking) One toy may be particularly popular	⇒
Whole body control	Sitting with support or for a few seconds alone Rolling over	Sitting steadily and pivoting to reach toys Some movement – shuffling, pushing up, rolling	⇒
Looking	Looking for dropped toys and at part of his body if it is touched Watching people and objects	Looks for and finds a toy if it is hidden under a cloth Recognizes familiar faces	⇒
Using hands	Holding things for a longer time and passing them from one hand to another Toys and any other objects may be put in his mouth	He plays using both hands His finger and thumb are used to pick up small objects	⇒
Listening and understanding	Turns his head towards a sound Showing interest in different sounds, e.g. loud/soft	He listens to conversation and responds when his name is said Imitates and produces new sounds	⇒
Communication	He seems to talk using babble and actions He can show excitement at mealtimes or when you go out	He plays "give and take" games He can babble using two syllables	⇒
Doing it myself	Holding a piece of toast to eat Learning what he looks like in a mirror	Finger feeds or attempts to hold a spoon He's displeased if thwarted	⇒

for these, the next little steps in his progress, so give him lots of extra claps and cuddles when he tries. Always remember to show him how pleased you are when he learns to do something by himself.

Slowly, almost imperceptibly, your baby's growing towards the next major change in his development – being on the move. His horizons are expanding fast. When you take him out for a walk or put him on a rug on the grass on a sunny day, he can see new things and try to reach them. Enjoy these times – they will pass all too quickly!

Watch out – everything he can reach will go straight into his mouth!

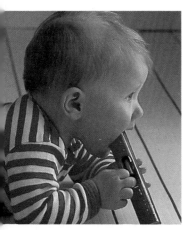

Baby's day

When your baby can sit, his day broadens to include playtimes as well as regular sleeping or eating times.

Playing safely

Set aside a play area for him where he can explore his new skills in safety. Put your precious things out of harm's way! Place a few toys on a tray on his playmat or chair; he is easily overwhelmed by too many playthings and won't be able to cope if a big box full of toys is put in front of him.

While your baby is practicing new skills, he can seem to be quite destructive. New things fascinate him; because he enjoys grabbing them, and might drop or throw them, it's important to make sure his play area is in a sensible place. The best place is often near the center of activity of the house, probably a part of the kitchen. Pretty nurseries at the top of the stairs will not be much used at this stage, however lovingly they have been thought out. He wants to be near you and see you, and you want to watch him.

Making the day fun

Use games to make routine activities more fun. Sing rhymes at bathtime, for example "rub a dub dub, three men in a tub." A baby quickly learns to associate certain

times of the day with having a good time. He'll start to look forward to diaper changes, bathtimes and mealtimes.

A relaxed routine can help

As well as having a routine at home, going out and seeing friends may be important to you both. Fitting such outings into the day is easier if he has a regular daytime nap and a reliable feeding pattern. Often mealtimes are long-drawn-out affairs as he plays with his food, fascinated by its color, texture, and taste. You may be in a hurry, however! Try giving him his own spoon and unbreakable bowl to play with, with a small quantity of food in it, while you give him his dinner from another bowl. In this way he can practice a skill and learn to use it without his whole meal going astray with very little being eaten.

Some people find the establishment of daily routines difficult, but they often help a baby to know where he stands and teach him to expect certain events and remember them. A routine may also help to make your life more settled so that you can set aside some time for yourself and for your partner. But some babies just do not want to fit into a strict routine and trying to force it will only make you feel frustrated.

Toys and playthings

Your baby will still enjoy playing with some of his early toys, but he'll benefit from some new ones to help him with his new skills.

Toys he can make work

An ideal toy for this age which he can watch and later pull towards him is a duck or caterpillar with moving parts. He may also be able to hold a musical box and pull the string to make it play. Give him toys that he can hold and make work: it may be one that squeaks when squeezed, or a drum he can thump. Either will hold your baby's attention, and encourage him to repeat his game. Revolving toys, too, will give him great pleasure. Toys which have parts that can be pushed out of sight and then pop up again can give hours of fun. Your baby may be fascinated by the fact that something can disappear and reappear.

Toys that won't roll away

As your baby cannot move very far, toys which stay within his reach are best. Dolls or other toys with rounded bases or on suction pads are a good idea. He can have great fun knocking them to and fro and they won't move too far away.

Exploring his toys

Your baby enjoys putting things to his mouth, not only because he wants to eat them, but because his mouth is a very sensitive place which can tell him a lot about this toy he's so interested in: is it hard, soft, cold, warm, solid? You can see him feeling the different textures of his toys and comparing one with another. He'll do this with other senses too, discovering that shaking a bell makes quite a different noise from banging a drum. Since his movements are not yet precise and may be quite erratic, it's important to place toys near him so he can touch them.

Toys to pick up and feel. Any toys which you buy at this stage should be easy to pick up. Cups which are easily held and which have shapes on the bottom to feel, spoons and pegs can all be enjoyed. Certain shapes are easier to pick up and hold than others; a sausage shape for example fits easily into a small hand. Your baby will still enjoy playing with a few objects strung across his chair – keys, pieces of paper and curtain rings, for example. They all feel interesting and make nice noises if touched or crumpled. But remember he will still pull them to his mouth!

A surprise box

With his increasing ability to pick up smaller objects, your baby will enjoy putting his hands inside a box to feel around and find a new toy. Your handbag is a paradise for him, but it's best kept out of reach. Find an old bag and fill it with harmless small things. Make a round hole in the top of a shoe box or cardboard box so that he can delve inside to reach some small objects: scraps of material, keys, plastic measuring spoons, etc. When he can pick up

Toys to buy

1. A ball or toy with moving parts mounted on a suction pad
2. Revolving toys – merry-go-rounds, activity centers, maypoles, etc.
3. Toys to bang – xylophone, drum, hammer, balls, pegs
4. A ball or small toy to push – a chime box with stick or a bounce-back doll
5. A book of rhymes or board books

Toys to make

1. A surprise box for finding and feeling playthings
2. A fabric "sausage" with a bell or buttons sewn on, made of different bits of material to touch
3. Saucepans and wooden spoons, an old cake tin, a plastic bottle with beans inside
4. Large light bricks, made of washable foam and covered with fabric

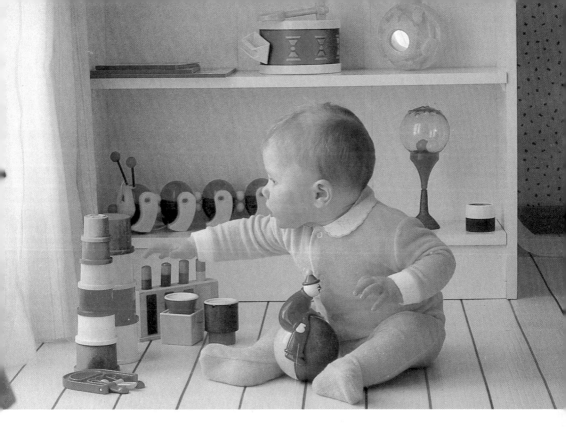

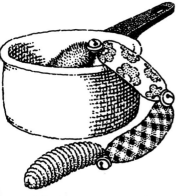

Now that she can sit, your baby will have great fun with toys that she can hold and work for herself.

even smaller objects, put a cracker or a raisin in the "magic box." Make sure none of the objects would do any harm if placed in his mouth.

Try hiding some of his things in a box and then showing them to him. Soon he'll want to look for himself to see what he can find.

Enjoying books and rhymes

Books continue to play an important part in his fun. He learns to listen to new games and is excited to see his toys or favorite cuddly object in a picture on a page. He will also enjoy listening to rhymes or short repetitive tunes. Slowly but surely his understanding is growing.

Games to play

From the start, babies love games, not only for sheer fun but also because playing games gives you and your baby an opportunity to enjoy one another's reactions as he tries out new skills.

Physical games

Your baby may enjoy quite physical games – being held under the arms and swung, clapping hands, a noisy rough-and-tumble. Play "pat-a-cake," take turns on a drum or play "hand over hand" – put one hand down, hold baby's hand over yours, let go, then put your hand on top of baby's. You may end up just clapping one hand on another, but he'll enjoy following whatever you do.

Gently help him to develop his new skills of balancing and sitting. Prop him up against a cushion then move it away and let him balance on his own. Be ready to catch him if he tumbles.

When he is on his tummy, hold a favorite toy above his head, just out of his reach; he will try to get it. Don't tease him; let him have the toy after a minute. In this way he's not only practicing a new skill but learning to enjoy a challenge.

<u>Gripping and grasping.</u> Holding and gripping a toy and then letting it go is typical behavior for a baby of this age. To help him grip, try pulling him gently backwards and forwards when he is sitting. He will hold on to your fingers, enjoying the movement, especially if you sing "Row the boat" at the same time! Be careful he does not fall backwards though; place a large pillow behind him to make a soft landing if he lets go of your hands unexpectedly. He may also enjoy trying to grasp dangling toys, or a musical box. Hold it just out of his reach for a moment so that he stretches for it before you give it to him.

Games with words

Developments in your baby's ability to talk to you are an important factor in games and

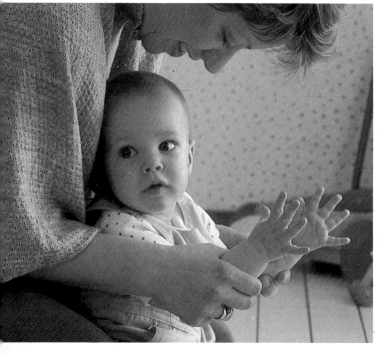

Make a game of teaching your baby to clap his hands.

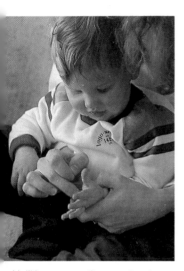

He'll love games, like round and round the garden, that involve words and movements.

play. He will almost certainly enjoy being carried around, having different objects pointed out to him and learning their names. He will revel in social contact and delight at games such as "round and round the garden" and "this little piggy."

Copying is fun

Copying you is a favorite game. Build a tower of beakers and knock it down, then watch him try to copy you. Rebuild the tower for him. Tentatively at first he will reach out and hit it, feeling huge-

Safety

Creating a safe environment for your baby depends on thinking ahead to prevent accidents. You can relax when you know he plays in safety. Watch out for the following:

- Your baby is at the stage when all objects are brought to his mouth. His toys should be clean, without sharp edges or breakable parts. Since he can reach out for things that excite his curiosity, keep objects like buttons and bottles of bleach or cleaning powder out of his way.
- Take care where you put him and do not turn away for too long. It is better for him to topple on to a cushion than a hard floor but once he has fallen he cannot regain his balance and play with his toys. If this happens he may become very distressed. As he is also leaning forward and reaching, his chair or playmat must be placed on the floor. Avoid the temptation of putting him on a table or not strapping him in his chair; he may fall and hurt himself badly.
- Most babies enjoy playing with sand and water, but be careful if older children are around. Sand thrown in a baby's eyes can do great harm and water in a paddling pool is dangerous to babies and toddlers alike. *Never* leave him sitting alone in even a few inches of water. Don't restrict your baby, but always make sure he is safe.
- Bathtime is another opportunity for new experiences. Be organized so that you can give baby all your attention. Make sure the water is the right temperature, keep one arm round him, leaving the other free to wash him, and make sure everything you need is comfortably within reach.

Many safety rules apply throughout childhood. The important thing is to be aware of children's limitations at the same time as helping them extend their horizons.

ly pleased with himself when the beakers roll all over the floor. This game shows him new skills, such as making things balance and putting them in order according to size. He's not ready to try this himself yet but he likes watching you do it.

Now I can move

Whether he's crawling, shuffling on his bottom or walking round the furniture, once your baby's on the move he'll be into everything and exploring everywhere.

At around nine or ten months, your baby starts to move around by himself, and a whole world opens up to him. He can get to where he wants under his own steam. Because he can also reach and hold on to things more easily, he is able to grab what he wants. However he gets around – by crawling, rolling, shuffling along on his bottom or stepping around the furniture – his progress will be speedy. No longer will you be able to leave the room to fetch something and find him in the same place when you come back. The room is far too interesting for him to stay sitting still for long; exploring is a new game.

Although moving about will give him a lot of pleasure and excitement, it can lead him into danger too. He can get to places which were out of his reach before. Stairs, fires, outlets, household cleaners, low cupboards with glass or sharp objects inside – these are some of the things which will now attract him, and from which he must be protected.

Many other changes are happening during these months. One you may be looking out for is your baby's first words. Around the time of his first birthday it should be clear what these words are. It is a time of rapid change; he is preparing for toddlerhood.

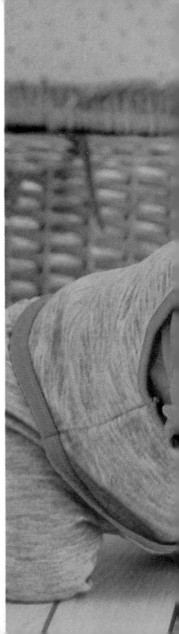

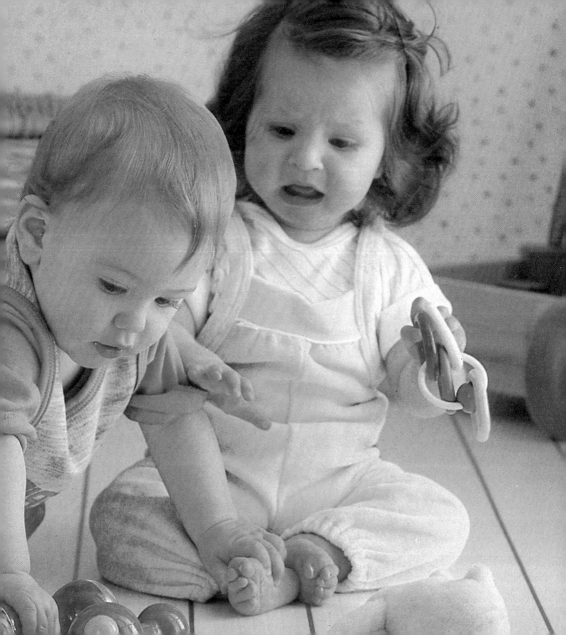

Skills of the baby on the move

When sitting still and playing no longer satisfies your baby, his efforts turn to finding some means of moving to get the things he wants.

Wanting to explore

At first he may only be able to turn around and reach behind him. In time he'll want to reach further and may get very cross when his struggles don't get him very far. Early attempts to move can be encouraged in a number of ways. Rolling a ball or putting a fascinating toy just out of his reach may tempt him to move towards it. Opening a cupboard or drawer which contains interesting but safe-to-touch objects is another encouragement to him to come over and have a look inside. If you get down to *his* level and show him the objects he'll want to join in even more.

Your baby won't start moving until his body is ready for it, no matter what inducements you provide, so don't force it or be concerned if he takes a little longer than some other babies to get moving. He'll start at the right time for him.

Different ways of moving

There are a number of ways in which your baby can get around and he may use one or a combination of methods. He may roll over and over or shuffle on his bottom until he reaches a low piece of furniture such as a chair or coffee table which he can use to pull himself to his feet. In time he'll start to make steps holding on to the furniture. Crawling often starts by pulling himself forward with his hands, moving his tummy along the floor. Quickly he progresses to using his hands and knees. Crawling can be quite hard-wearing on the knees, so protect them by putting him in trousers or dungarees, especially if he is going to try out his new skill in the yard!

It will take quite a lot of effort from your baby when he first starts moving, but as soon as he gets it right crawling or shuffling will seem second nature to him. Soon he may be attempting to get up and down a low step dividing one room from another, and may show interest in clambering up your bottom stairs. These are the beginnings of climbing, but it will be a while yet before he can manage to get on to a chair or bed without help.

Pulling himself up

When your baby first starts pulling himself up on to his feet, he can't get down again and may fall back with a bump. By standing up, holding on, he gradually

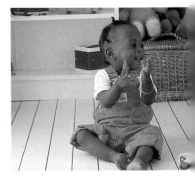

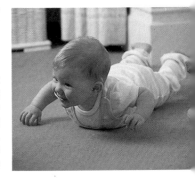

Once she's learned how, she'll clap at any and every opportunity (top). Learning to crawl takes a lot of effort but it's fun trying (above).

learns to balance himself on his feet so that later, when he is stronger, he will be ready to stand on his own. If you take his hands in yours and move slowly backwards you can help him take his first steps.

Toys that can help

A baby walker trolley, with an upright handle to prevent it tipping over, is an aid to walking. He can also use it to push around his favorite toys. Until he can pull himself up you will need to help him with this toy. Baby walkers with a small canvas seat suspended in a frame on small wheels can also be useful as they open up the possibilities of movement. However, they don't allow him to practice pulling himself on to his feet nor balancing on his own.

Using his hands

Your baby may be so absorbed by his new means of exploring that his progress in other areas slows down, but he'll still be inching forward with other activities. His handling of objects, once something of a hit-and-miss affair, is more deliberate. His eyesight has improved, so things catch his attention even if they are not right in front of him. He can reach out purposefully for a toy you offer him, look carefully at it and turn it over to inspect each part. If he drops it, he'll watch where it falls or rolls.

No longer does he scoop small things up into the palm of his hand but gradually starts picking them up between his thumb and first finger. He may be fasci-

nated by picking up small crumbs off a dish or pulling at threads on a carpet or blanket. He will still put things into his mouth at this age so this kind of play can be very trying. To let him practice using his hands, attach a favorite toy to a piece of string so he can pull it along or provide him with some pullalong toys. Soon he starts poking and pointing at things with his fingers and uses both hands more efficiently.

Copying you

Your baby loves to copy actions you've made for him. He may now take the lead in "peek-a-boo," spontaneously wave bye-bye and clap his hands when he is pleased. To start with he may not always do these things at the right time – he just enjoys the actions – but soon he'll work out you wave when it's time to go.

Learning to let go

Your baby may offer things to you, just as you held out your hand to offer things to him, but without realizing that he has to let go of an object in order to give it. This inability to release something from his grasp can also be seen when he first tries to place one block on another. Very likely he will not be able to remove his hand from the top block without knocking it off. He'll return to the challenge of blocks again.

Doing things for himself

Your baby will now be taking a greater part in many everyday activities. If you are putting on his coat he can transfer a toy he's holding from one hand to the other in order to put his arm through the sleeve, and he may really push his arm into the sleeve rather than let you pull it on for him. These actions are a good example of how different skills combine to make further achievements. He has *understood* what is required, *remembered* and *copied* what he has seen before, and has the *control* over his arms to carry out part of the action himself.

Holding his own cup or bottle when drinking, or feeding himself fingers of toast or slices of fruit, are things he is probably very good at by now. He may enjoy the challenge of using a spoon but will not be quite so skillful with it as he is with his fingers.

Talking and understanding

Your greatest delight will probably come from hearing your baby's first words. Usually they are the names of things he knows well or words he often hears you use. He has probably been able to understand a good deal for a while now and will have learned the difference between angry and pleased tones of voice.

NOW I CAN MOVE (around 9 to 12 months)

	moving →	exploring →	walking →
Making sense of the world	He can choose toys and play in a deliberate way	His whole world is expanding He's now into everything!	
Whole body control	He sits steadily for long periods, may reach and turn around He may be starting to move back or forwards	He pulls himself up on the furniture He may take some steps holding on	
Looking	Looks and smiles at himself in the mirror He can watch others from quite a long way away	He can find familiar places or toys in his own house He watches events going on for a long time, e.g. cars moving, dad washing up, birds pecking	
Using his hands	Using his finger and thumb to pick things up Likes holding small objects	He enjoys scribbling, throwing, taking things out of containers, pulling and pushing small toys, or poking and pointing	
Listening	He listens to and copies a greater number of sounds He may move to find out where noises are coming from	He enjoys listening to rhymes, music Short repetitive stories may hold his interest too	
Communicating	He babbles or shouts for attention He will show affection Shakes his head for "no"	Shows the beginnings of some recognizable words Points, waves bye-bye Joins in simple songs, e.g. "pat-a-cake"	
Looking after himself	He's using his fingers, he may help to hold a spoon at mealtimes Shows what he likes and dislikes	He continues to do more things for himself He holds his own cup Helps in dressing He can get the things he wants, e.g. his cup, toys, etc.	

Baby's day now that he's on the move

By this time you and your baby have probably settled into some kind of regular daily pattern, of which going out forms a particularly important part. His gurgles and shouts may show you how pleased he is if you point to moving things like cars, trees, water or people as he sits in the carriage or stroller. His restless curiosity makes it difficult for him to sit in one place for too long, however, and long shopping trips may not be easy!

Eating, sleeping and bathtime will have settled into a routine that meets his needs and suits the rest of the family. Lunchtime, for example, may have to be fitted in between his naps, and to suit an older child returning from morning playgroup or nursery school. As your baby will increasingly want to do things for himself, eating his meals can take a long time. What he likes and doesn't like to eat and drink will be clearly shown.

Less time is now taken up by his naps. Perhaps he has just one long sleep in the day, with one or two shorter naps or periods of quiet play. As he is using up more energy, naps and rest times are still important. Even if you are out at times when he's usually rest-

ing, try to settle him down for a nap as it can help prevent irritable patches later on. He may just doze in the stroller or carriage.

A "cuddly"

By this time you will know if your baby has attached himself to a particular toy or object, such as a piece of blanket, cloth diaper, cloth or soft toy, which he likes to clutch for comfort when he is tired or upset. Some babies will suck a pacifier or their thumb at these times as well. Maybe your baby does not have a cuddly, but if he does it is very important to him, the one thing you mustn't forget when you go on a journey, especially if you're going away from home overnight. Cleaning the cloth or toy can cause a great upset so think about buying an identical one at an early stage to take the place of the other when necessary.

Shyness

At this stage, too, you may notice a change in the way he reacts to others. While once he accepted all other adults and was friendly to whoever talked to him or picked him up, now he may be less willing to acknowledge strangers, clinging to you and hiding his face if they talk to him. He may also be wary in strange or new places. Even with people he knows he may hesitate a little

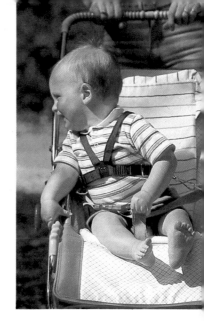

There's so much to look around at.

before smiling at them. Some of this shyness comes about because he is now very sure of who and what he knows. He has learned who he is and will smile when he sees himself in the mirror. He's also learning about possessions – which is his cup, chair or brush. His awareness that he can do so many new things for himself affects his relationship with you. He may realize he needs you less now to do certain things, but he still needs you in so many other ways. Give him the confidence to progress further by your reassurance and patience.

Toys and playthings

An amazing world has now opened up to your baby. Everything in the house or garden will attract him. Food, waste paper baskets, shoes and boxes are playthings to your baby just as much as any toy you buy. Though he may still be entertained by what goes on around him, now he wants to join in too. Playing near you is still important. Give him a low cupboard in the kitchen (make sure it's out of your way so you don't trip over him) and put safe but interesting things in it for him to get out while you get on with other things.

Toys he'll want to follow

Before your baby could move, toys that rolled out of his reach probably made him very frustrated. These same toys now encourage him to move. A brightly colored ball or a toy which rolls along making a clattering or jangling noise may particularly tempt him. Pushing a small toy on wheels past him may have the same effect. A wooden car or truck moves slower than a plastic or metal one so it will be easier for him to follow, and if it has a driver or passenger which comes out this makes it even more interesting. Toys like this will be used again and again in different games as he grows.

Finding out about things

Exploration is the name of his favorite game. The toys and objects that his little hands and fingers can get into may be as popular as those encouraging him to move. A cardboard box, saucepan or child's bucket are all good containers to explore. You can put things in them such as clothespins, a bunch of keys, empty spools or some of his small toys. This will make him want to delve inside and get them out, though he will not yet be so good at putting them back. A sorting box, with a lid which can be easily removed, can be used in a similar way.

Making things work

He is now much busier with his hands and using them to find out what he can make his toys do. Small push-and-pull-along toys are satisfying and baby toys can be used in new ways. Tying a short piece of cord to a rattle makes a simple pull-along toy. He may be able to pull the string on a dangling mobile; a wooden man or animal whose limbs "jump" out when a string is pulled gives a lot of fun. The dial of a toy telephone or moving parts on rattles also encourage him to use his fingers to explore.

A jack-in-the-box or a pop-up toy is exciting and helps him

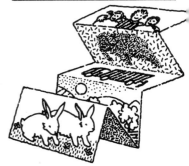

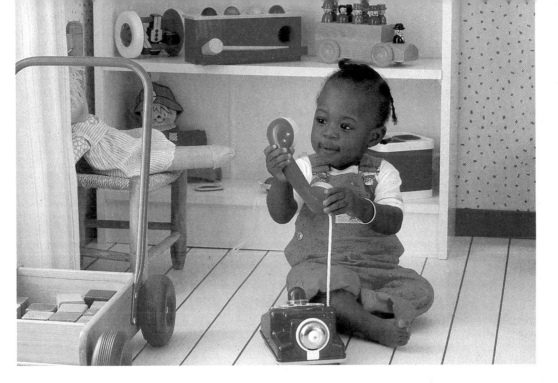

Toys that can be explored and used are a source of fun now.

realize "if I do this, that happens." Place your hand over his while you close the lid or push the button. Some children of this age can be a bit frightened of toys like this and may prefer a little merry-go-round or swingboat.

New skills and old favorites

Some toys and games need two hands to make them work – playing with a ball, picking up a large box or container, holding and turning the pages of a book – all of these your baby can cope with now. New toys may attract him but by now it's clear which are his favorite playthings. A scrapbook of photographs of himself or his family or pictures of everyday objects is easy to do together. The pictures can be changed as he gets older.

Toys for his second year

For your baby's first birthday choose presents with an eye to what he will be doing in the next few months. Crayons, a bag or tub of bricks, a pull-along toy, big shapes which easily fit together, a sorting box, a simple jigsaw with knobs on the pieces to make it easy to lift and look under – all of these he can play with now and use again as he grows. Larger toys such as a sit-on tricycle, push wagon or toy carriage are also good buys. Saving some of his birthday or Christmas gifts to introduce later when he is not well or if you have to stay indoors is a good idea and prolongs the enjoyment of getting new things.

Games to play

Your baby will enjoy games that let him try out new ways of moving; push him in a baby swing, sit with him on your lap on a merry-go-round or seesaw. Riding in the seat of a supermarket cart can also be fun. Pointing to different items on the shelves or letting him hold one of the unbreakable packets can turn shopping into a game.

Bathtime fun

At bathtime, he may enjoy splashing the water vigorously with his arms and legs, making his floating toys bob up and down. Since he can sit steadily, his hands are free to play with his bath toys. Filling up and emptying containers may fascinate him, although he cannot pour water carefully yet. Pulling him through the water on his tummy or back by holding him under the arms may cause many gurgles of laughter and give him the delicious sensation of water moving all around him.

Copying and learning

Imitating you, still a favorite game, is also a way of showing you what he likes to do. He can copy with his mouth and with his hands . He can smack his lips, cough or say "brrr." He can wave, clap his hands or bang them on a table. He may start off a game of

"peek-a-boo" with you by hiding behind a chair or door and peeking out. He's very interested too in looking at himself and may stare, smile or offer a toy to the reflection of himself in a mirror.

Letting things go

Games in which he offers things to you and you give them back

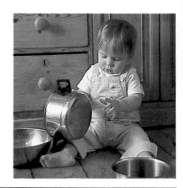

Ordinary household objects make a lot of noise and can be great fun.

Safety

Your active baby won't stay long in one place: he'll be off exploring everywhere and everything.

- Do not leave him, even for a few seconds, on a bed or on his changing mat on a high surface. He can easily roll or fall off.
- He may wriggle and strain to get out of his high chair or stroller. Make it a rule always to use a harness to strap him in.
- Rooms which were once safe for him to play in are now full of dangers. Electrical outlets to poke fingers in, steps or stairs to explore and climb, breakable or sharp objects to pull off low shelves or tables, are all possible playthings to him. Use outlet covers, built or buy a stairgate, and move ornaments out of sight, to prevent accidents and reassure you that he is safe at play.
- He may still be taking things to his mouth. Make sure sharp objects or those small enough to swallow are not left on the floor. Toys need to have non-toxic paint and should not break if he throws or bites them. Are there any poisonous plants in your garden? Those bright red berries or shiny leaves could give him a nasty stomach ache, or worse. Stay with him so that you can keep a watchful eye on him without stopping him exploring.
- A playpen with a few favorite toys inside can be useful though he'll get restless if left in the playpen for too long.
- Make sure anything he can use to pull himself up is sturdy enough to take his weight.

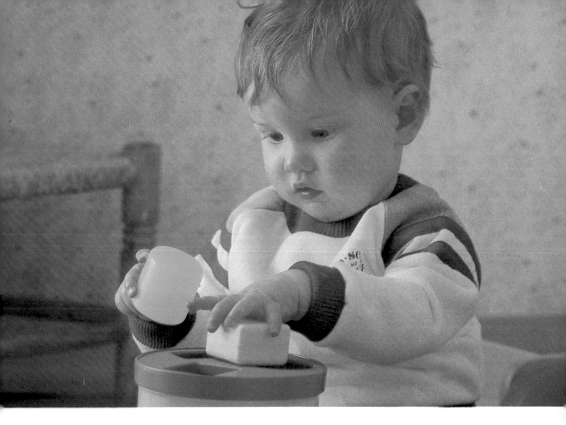

allow him to learn about sharing and joining in. They help him understand what you want him to do at certain times. Rolling a ball to and fro shows him he can play with a toy even if he is not holding on to it. Playing "swap," where you exchange toys, is another simple game that helps him learn to let go of an object.

Exploring games
Some games are experiments, ways of finding out about things: whether two objects fit together, for example. He may find out that a small ball fits into a large cup but not a large ball into a small cup. Banging a spoon on different tins or containers tells him which makes the most interesting or loudest noise. His enjoyment of putting something inside a box or under a cup and taking it out and putting it in again is teaching

First tries at sorting can be puzzling. him that the object is still there even though he cannot see it clearly. Hiding a small toy under a cloth and seeing if he can find it takes the game a step further. Make it easy at first by letting part of the toy stick out of the cloth. Talk about the game as you play it. Your baby will soon begin to repeat some games on his own.

Now I can walk

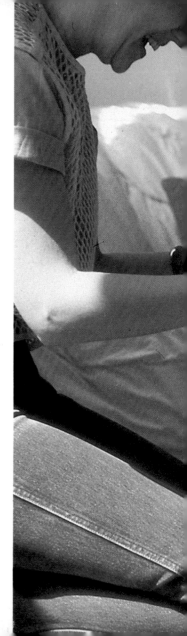

His first steps are a great thrill and he gradually becomes more confident and independent, enjoying larger toys and games with other children.

As your baby grows into a toddler you'll take pride in his increased confidence and his pleasure in doing things for himself. He can walk and perhaps he has started to talk; but he still needs you, the warmth you can give him and the security your relationship provides. From this he can reach out into a busy world.

Most babies start to walk at any time from 10 to 18 months. Your baby's everyday moods, ups and downs, will affect how quickly he acquires new skills like these. Don't compare his progress with that of other toddlers and try not to worry when a friend compares your toddler to another; we are all different! Your baby is mastering new actions all the time. His babbling leads on to words; he may try to put a hat on a doll or put your shoes on or feed himself. Every day he is learning and enjoying your company, putting down the foundations for the next little steps in his progress.

Skills of the toddler

When your baby first learns a new skill, such as walking, he will be absorbed by it and excited by the extra freedom it gives him. As he discovers new pleasures, old ones are discarded along with baby toys. Looking back over the

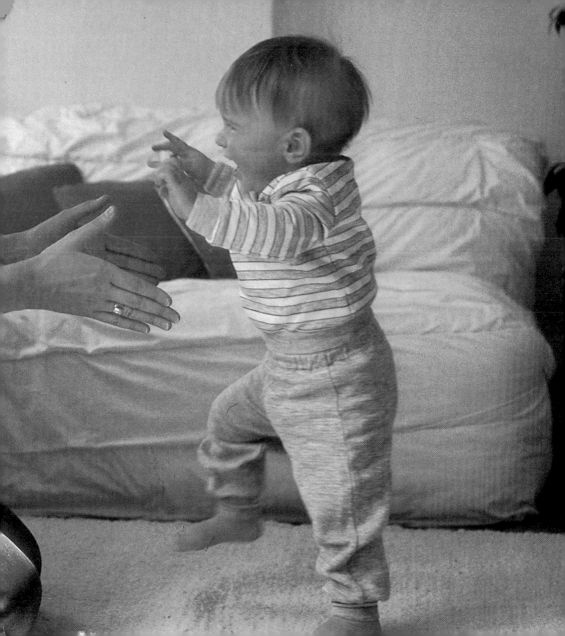

What the toddler can do

weeks you'll be astonished by the amount he's learned.

There's a certain satisfaction in writing down the stages your toddler passes through as you watch them happen. On the way to becoming a competent walker, he moves around holding on to furniture, then reaches out between two pieces of furniture and then takes his first steps. As his confidence grows, he may edge away from the furniture and take three or four steps towards you. Day by day his confidence and balance increase until he can walk alone across a room and even pull a toy behind him.

Walking and running

Some babies take off very quickly when learning to walk, others make a spurt and then stop. Illness or a fall will naturally make him more cautious, but these are only temporary setbacks. As his balance improves he'll enjoy outdoor games more. Most children try to kick a ball, some even before they can walk! Soon he may be running after the ball and kicking it to you. The speed with which he progresses in walking is probably the most distinctive feature of this age.

Building and sorting

Your toddler will also be able to do more with his hands. Building towers of blocks or placing hoops

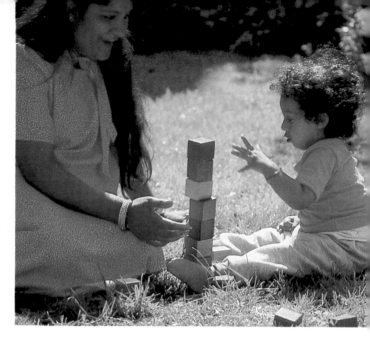

Your toddler will soon be building a tower of blocks – wobbly at first!

on the pole of a stacking toy are favorite activities for a 12-18 month old. He's finding out all about shapes which stack easily, and he can hold small objects and put them down carefully. He can fit some simple shapes into matching holes. The first shape may be a circle, as there are no edges which will catch, and later on he'll place a square or triangular shape through a hole in a box. He will soon learn how to get them out once they have been put in, in order to play again.

Experiments and independence

By the time your toddler is 18 months old you may have forgotten the relative peace you had when he was crawling! Now that he can turn knobs and taps, fill containers with water – and spill it – he'll be up to no end of tricks. He is constantly experimenting. You'll have to watch him carefully in this time of growing independence. He can play by himself for short spells; turn the pages of a book; open his toy cupboard, find a toy and take it out. He is learning to choose and is gaining confidence in his own choices. Where once you had to do every-

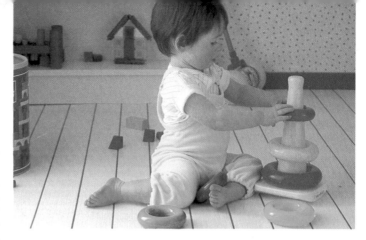

thing, now you must stand back and indulge your toddler's intense desire to do as much as possible for himself.

Using his imagination

While some baby toys will be permanently outgrown, other favorite toys may be revived in different ways. You'll see that his imagination is developing as his other skills increase. Hammering the pegs on a board will be extended to using tools "like daddy does," or banging a drum. He is learning to use implements to do some specific task. He can now sweep the floor, as you do, and try to wipe up – he wants to try everything that's going.

Remembering and learning

Learning from experience and remembering what is familiar is part of your toddler's progress. He recognizes shapes and objects in a jigsaw puzzle and can see how they fit. At first he may try to put the piece in upside down, but he knows where it goes.

First scribbles

It is about this time that your toddler is ready to enjoy his first set of crayons. Stubby crayons are best to start with, and it helps to stick the paper to his highchair or a tabletop with tacks or tape. It is a difficult set of skills he is trying to master; he has to hold a crayon, push it against the paper

and move it. Sometimes holding your hand over his makes these early steps easier.

He will enjoy being creative, scribbling over a whole page or just in one corner. It is quite amazing how much he can teach himself. Encourage him and praise all his products.

Learning to talk

Children vary enormously in the age at which they say their first words. You can help immeasurably by talking to him and paying attention to his responses. Eventually you will see signs that his understanding is increasing, he is listening, following what you are saying and doing things before you do! He will point, pull at you or grimace, as well as making some noises in answer to yours. These are all milestones on the road to speech. Many toddlers begin by naming familiar people

Learning about shapes, sizes, color and order is all tremendous fun.

or objects: "daddy," "car," "shoe" or "juice." Later on he may be able to say "more" or "gone" at mealtimes and tell you what he is doing: "bang," "jump." It is essential to listen to him; if his utterings are unclear, say the word again for him, but never let him feel he's got it wrong. He's trying very hard, and that's what matters. He cannot produce all the sounds in the word at first, but he needs to hear them. P, B, D and G (as in garden) are the easiest sounds for him to say; S or F will come later. Giving your toddler a lot of attention, praising his efforts, and asking him to do simple things with you will encourage him to talk and that ability opens up a whole new world for you all.

NOW I CAN WALK (around 12 to 18 months)

	walking ➡	constructing ➡	chatting ➡
Making sense of the world	Beginning to see what his toys will do His main play is with construction toys	He's building up a greater understanding of world – inside and outside, up and down, naughty and good	➡
Whole body control	Taking a few steady steps Kneeling, stooping, climbing stairs	Trotting around, carrying or pulling a toy Kicking a ball, balancing briefly on one leg	➡
Looking	Looking at detail in picture books, and now he's placing a ball in a hole He can follow a toy if it is moved quickly across a table	He can match several shapes (especially ○ and □) in a shape sorter or do a simple jigsaw Pointing to distant objects	➡
Using his hands	Movements are more precise He's picking up small things with his thumb and finger, turning pages of book, banging xylophone	His actions are more constructive He's building a tower, pouring water, or turning knobs Scribbling	➡
Listening	He participates in noisy play, e.g. "singing" and dancing to music Carrying out simple instructions, e.g. "where are your shoes?"	He recognizes and he may seek familiar noises (e.g. door bell, fire engine) Understanding more complex instructions	➡
Communicating	He may "jabber" and use a few words Increased facial expression – pouting and showing excitement	When he asks for things he may use both gestures and words, he may point to named parts of body He may be using more words	➡
Looking after himself	He can manage food and drink He takes his hat or socks off	Helps his mother to wash and dress himself Maneuvering himself confidently around house and garden Plays alone for a short time	➡

The toddler's day

During your toddler's second year, he will often want to be involved in what you're doing, so much so that it can seem to take hours to do things like getting him ready to go out! Routines are important now if you want to have certain times when he can do what he wants to do or show you new games, while learning that at other times it's necessary to co-operate and fit in.

As your toddler grows up your life becomes busier and it can become more difficult to find times to play and relax and enjoy his company. This is still very important: if he sees that you are enjoying his company and he is able to enjoy yours he will be more co-operative at other times.

Copying what you're doing

His enjoyment of games and sense of achievement as he learns to do things give him added confidence. Copying you is still one of his favorite amusements, so involve him whenever you can. He can stand on a small stool near you as you shell the peas, or have his own washing up bowl near your sink, to wash his plastic cups or spoons; let him empty the washing machine with you and help put things away.

Helping him to play

Too many toys can be confusing

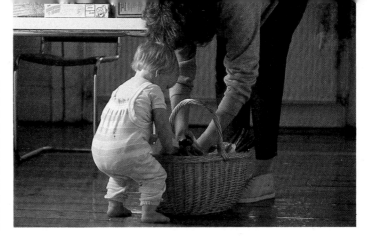

Your toddler loves being helpful!

and lead to frustration. Put some in his bedroom and bring a few downstairs. He will need enough to choose from but not so many that he can't decide. Watch him to see if he is overwhelmed and just flitting from one toy to another. Put a few different ones out each day, as well as some smaller ones like cars and puzzles and a few old favorites. Introduce a new toy occasionally.

Put your toddler's toys where he can easily find the ones he wants. The toys at the back of the cupboard are less often played with because they can't be reached. If you put toys in stacking boxes which can be lifted off or in drawers which can be pulled out, you may encourage him to find them and play with them. Organizing his toys is an important way in which you can help him to play.

Talking and listening

Talking and listening to him makes little demand on you but is an important part of his progress. Tell him the names of everything you see, then listen to him trying out the words. You may notice how he starts with one or two words, then maybe forgets them and learns some new ones, retaining favorite words which he continues to use.

Going out

A daily outing is a good thing for both of you, especially if it involves the company of other children and their parents. A mother-and-toddler group is an ideal place for him to try out new, perhaps bigger toys and for both of you to make new friends. He is learning to find pleasure in his own company and with others.

Toys and playthings

When your toddler gains confidence on his feet he may enjoy "push- and pull-along" toys.

Push- and pull-along toys

Most toddlers manage push-along toys first, possibly because it is easier to balance pushing a toy along. The first big toys for pushing need to be very steady. Make sure the toy doesn't move too easily and run away with him; generally wooden examples are more reliable in this respect. You can make your own pull-along toy; a can or long plastic container with rice, a peg or an old key in it would make a lovely sound. A short piece of string may be better than a long one, and safer. Choose a low, wide container with some weight to it.

His growing imagination can be seen in the different uses to which he puts his toys. His block wagon now transports toys or doubles as a stroller or wheelbarrow. He'll sit on a pull-along car and pretend to be the driver.

Some toys now take on a different role. A favorite doll or teddy bear may be treated like one of the family – dressed, bathed, fed, put in a stroller for outings, and even told off!

Building and stacking toys

Twelve to eighteen months is the age when toys to build with become popular. As well as beakers and blocks he might enjoy a stacking toy which is shaped as a pyramid, so the large shapes fit first and then the smaller ones. While a young toddler will be happy to play with just a few blocks to hold and stack, as he gets older his more adventurous attempts at building and his budding imagination, call for a bag or tub of blocks.

There are many toys which encourage him to find out how things fit together and can be combined to make simple structures. As he grows older you can add the extra features which stretch his imagination: farmyard animals, cars and airplanes.

Stringing

Some toddlers enjoy trying to string beads or blocks. The blocks are brightly colored and easy for him to hold, but at first you may need to hold your hand over his to help him put them on the string; eventually he'll be able to do this by himself. It is important that the hole in the middle is large and easily seen and that the string is of stiff plastic or he'll get despondent and give up.

Toys to interest your child

As at each stage, toddlers vary as to when they master certain skills and which toys they want to play with. If yours enjoys turning knobs, maybe a toy which unscrews or has to be wound up will prove to be successful. If he enjoys hammering, get him a tool bench or xylophone. If he enjoys putting bits together, a puzzle may be his favorite. If he enjoys music there are a large variety of simple musical instruments to choose from – a piano, a drum or tambourine – or even a simple wind-up record player. Toys like these will be used for ages.

Messy play

Stimulate his imagination in as many ways as you can. Give him different materials to play with: sand, water, playdough, paint and crayons. He'll be fascinated by the different textures and will chat to himself as he plays. He may begin to make things or copy you, filling beakers with wet sand and baking "pretend cakes"; water may be used for watering the garden or for washing faces. Bathtime is a great time for water play, of course, as well as one when you can both relax.

A large sit-on toy

At about 18 months, you may think of buying your toddler a large toy so that he can explore new ways of moving and climbing. Since many of these toys are expensive, it's best to let him try out one or two at a mother-and-toddler group. A sit-on bike or a

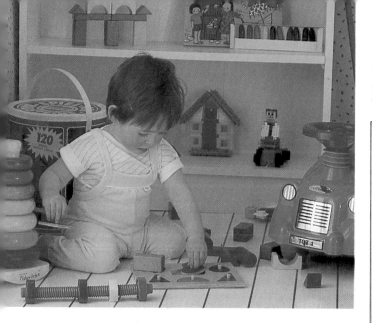

Toys the toddler will enjoy

Toys for building, stacking, fitting and stringing are all fun as your toddler grows more skillful with her hands.

Toys you can buy

1. Blocks – as many as possible
2. Sorting boxes. Simple ones (with O □ and ◁ shapes) are the best to buy
3. Simple puzzles with knobs on the pieces to make it easy to pull them out
4. A sit-on trike or car, small toy stroller or baby buggy, wheelbarrow
5. Crayons
6. Books – especially those with simple repetitive stories

Toys to make

1. A large cardboard box can be used as a sit-in car or boat. It can be turned upside down as a table, or even a miniature house
2. A pull-along toy
3. Playdough. This can be made from

    2 teaspoons cooking oil

    2 cups flour

    ½ cup salt

    then enough water to make it like real pastry

    coloring – powder paint

It can be stored in a refrigerator for a week or so
4. Things to string – curtain rings, keys, cotton reels, etc.

car pushed along by his feet may be a very good buy.

Enjoying books and songs

Looking at books begins to play a larger part in his day. At first their main function lies in introducing new words to him and letting him see how everyday objects are shown in a picture. Then they show him unfamiliar things, such as animals he will one day see at a zoo or games he can play on the beach on holiday. Music and songs always delight children at every stage of their development. Listening to a record of rhymes or to your voice singing is a source of great pleasure. Many toddlers at this age enjoy stories and rhymes which repeat themselves and have hand actions.

While this is a time for letting him play as he wants to, he looks to you for new ideas.

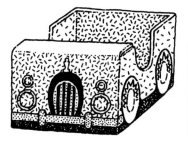

47

Games to play

Making a time during the day just for games is always a good idea, but the best games are often those which come out of everyday events like getting dressed, putting the shopping away, fetching things for you, or bathtime. If you turn these routines into play most of the day becomes one long game, and all activities are opportunities for him to learn to do things with you and follow what you say.

Hiding games

Even if he is not speaking, he is understanding more and more. The familiar game of hiding one or two toys under a cloth and then saying to him "find the bus" (or car, or doll) will help him to talk. He will be pleased if you repeat the game, laughing or pulling the cloth from you. Learning to anticipate things will also encourage him to use sounds. He may be nodding and shaking his head for "yes" and "no," or even saying "no." Another game could involve hiding a favorite toy, one he'll really want to find, and saying – "is it in the box?" – "no." "Is it in your crib?" – "no." "It's in the cupboard!"

Playing with other children

Most toddlers become aware of other children at this age, though he may not join in with them and will want you there as well. When he is walking steadily, he may like to join a small group to play ring-around-the-rosy, musical games or dancing. He will soon be copying the actions and be listening for the right tune. At first, he plays alongside other children that he meets, then gets the confidence to join in a little. Being there with him in the game gives him the boost he needs.

Games which encourage him to make noises or show you pictures may be popular. Making animal noises is great fun and he'll quickly learn how to meow like a cat or grunt like a pig.

Ring-around-the-rosy is fun and games like these encourage children to play together (below). Your child may need time to get used to a toy like a sit-on bike (right).

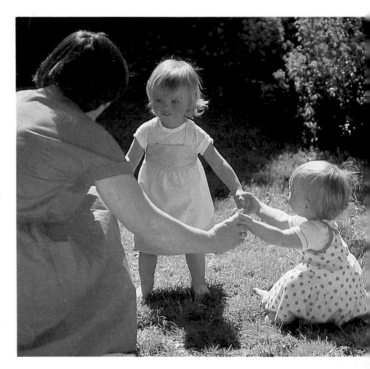

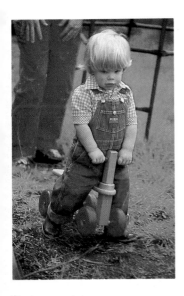

Playing outdoors

His ability to play more purposefully with a ball can be great fun. Dropping it and trundling after it are as good as catching it. He can get the ball, bring it and offer it for you to throw. Try kicking it to him; though he can't stop it yet, he may still try to kick it himself. You can play this indoors with a soft foam ball, not a balloon, which may burst.

Make the most of your local park, especially if it has a playground. Feeding the ducks, splashing in puddles and jumping in leaves are all great games for the toddler.

Safety

Your mobile toddler c̶ ̶ ̶ ̶ ̶es, turn knobs or taps and climb stairs. It is import̶ ̶ ̶ ̶explore and play safely.

- Your toddler's play̶ ̶ ̶ded to include the whole house. Since yo̶ ̶ ̶ ̶ ̶all the time you must ensure that there are ̶ ̶ ̶ ̶g in wait for him. His balance is at first unsteady̶ ̶ ̶not be able to manage steps. Use staircases ̶ ̶ ̶ ̶sary. Keep outside doors firmly closed to avoid f̶ ̶ ̶ ̶e steps. Don't leave bits and pieces lying arou̶ ̶ ̶p. Rugs and loose carpets on polished floors sho̶ ̶ ̶ ̶n with non-slip underlay.
- M̶ ̶ ̶ ̶no glass that can break at his level – for ̶ ̶ ̶panel in a door.
- ̶ ̶ ̶come downstairs safely, backwards as if climbing ̶ ̶ ̶a ladder. Each time you come to the stairs in your house, show him how you turn round and come downstairs. At first he may appear bewildered or amused, but soon he will learn and do it himself. He may turn round and begin his backwards move a few feet away from the top of the stairs. His overcaution is amusing, but he's erring on the right side.
- If you live in an apartment, take care with balconies and windows, and use window gates. If you have to leave the room, put him in a playpen, if you have one, or another safe place.
- When you are out on the road, a harness can keep him safe until he learns all about pavements and cars.
- Reaching, poking and holding can also be exciting new games for him, but since he can now reach the stove and poke at outlets, he must be protected. A burner guard, socket plugs and door catches are all useful ways of making life safe for him.
- It is always important to listen out for him and know what he is up to. As he grows up he can turn faucets and open screwtops on bottles and containers. Leave the bathroom door shut to avoid scalds from the hot faucet. Bottles of bleach, chemicals, alcohol and even aftershave should be locked out of sight.
- If you use a car, get a car seat properly installed. You may find that a harness is useful again on public transport.

Now I can talk

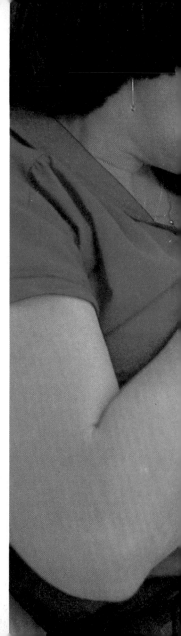

Your child has been understanding ▮▮▮▮ more and now he can express himself and re▮▮▮▮ his feelings known.

During his second year, your toddler is capable of a great deal – he can do lots of things for himself, tell you what he wants and is starting to decide how he wants to spend his day. The greatest change of all is that he understands you and is beginning to speak for himself. You may enjoy his attempts to do things for himself as much as he does. He may try to get his own lunch out of the refrigerator, or want to push his stroller in the park or along the pavement. He's experimenting with life and finding out what he can do. No longer content with exploring, he wants to play his part and join in.

I can chatter

Talking is one of the most complicated skills your child will ever learn. Think how the sounds your toddler makes, and his understanding, mature over his first two years. He can remember, think about, listen to and concentrate on a remarkable number of things. But he needs you to listen and respond to him, so he feels he has something worth saying.

First words

The chart "I can talk" shows the stages many children go through when learning to talk. At first his understanding is often better than his ability to speak. For example, he might get his plate just as you

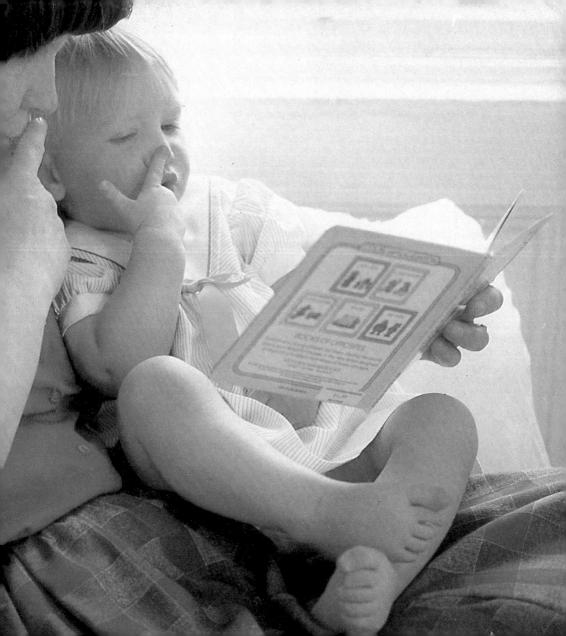

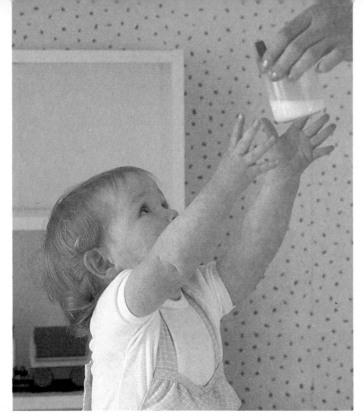

Now she can ask for what she wants.

thirsty, I need juice." Furthermore, he has to be able to move his mouth in the right way to make the word. Some toddlers may have achieved the first of these difficult steps (understanding, remembering and thinking) but may still be learning how to make the right sounds. Some may be shy and cautious and stay quiet in order not to make mistakes. But they'll be learning all the time.

Some children seem to use single words a great deal during their first months of "talk"; others tend to babble, with words mixed up in it. A toy telephone is fun for him at this stage.

Joining words together

As your toddler begins to join words together ("daddy car," "my shoes") it's easier for you to know exactly what he wants and needs. Two words can, however, be used to mean several different things; "daddy car" may mean "there's daddy's car," "daddy's car is outside, he's home," or "there's a car the same as daddy's." As he can say more, his exact meaning will be clearer. He will always enjoy seeing you respond to his words. Expand on what he says, make more of it – "yes, daddy is home, his car is outside."

Listening and learning

When he's learning to talk, it is

say to him "I must cook lunch." Though he may not be using words, your reaction, the fact that you understand, is all important.

When you are talking to your child it is important to have his attention. If he is directly looking at you he has every chance of understanding you; this is especially important if he has had lots

of colds which could affect his hearing at times. He may also find it easier if at first you point to the toy you are talking about or bring it to him. Don't bombard him with too much information at once. Your instructions to him need to be short and simple.

When he says his first words he has learned to listen to you, remembered a name – it may be "juice" – and had to think "I'm important that he feels you want to know what he has to say. At first his sounds will be incomplete and his grammar faulty, but if he is told to "say it properly" he may stop trying to say anything at all. He will learn what is right simply by listening to you and your conversations with other people.

If he says "mummy-go-wings," for example you could reply "yes, of course we can go to the swings." He knows you understand him and will try the words again. Some sounds are more difficult for all toddlers to say than others. For many months he may have trouble if a word has an "s," "ch,"

"sh," or "th" in it. Other mistakes he may make are forming the past tense by adding "ed" ("He goed") or making all plurals by adding an "s" ("foots"). By listening to you, he'll get it right.

Looking through the steps on the chart may give you ideas on how to encourage him to use new words. An example of this may be a game to encourage him to use verbs as well as nouns, and to use them together. Use the different activities of his favorite teddy bear to teach him this. Teddy can be washed, be dressed, fed and cuddled. Play "what's teddy doing?", or, better still, "Simon says." In this way he will soon learn to listen to verbs and may begin to use them. When looking at books with him, point out pictures of people doing things.

When you go out, you may wish your child would "show off" his new skills. But children rarely perform and toddlers can be very strong-willed. The best thing is to stand back; then he might relax and start to talk. But the chances are he won't. You may also find that at first not only will you have to act as interpreter but you may also have to stop people from correcting him. Tell them that many children say "bup" for "cup" at first, or "gog" for "dog"

Talking	Understanding
Saying first words	– comes when called – pointing to some of his toys – follows simple instructions (where is your cup; give it to me; show me) – points to some parts of his body (nose, hair)
Using 5 or more names (car, cup, dog) Says "no" May say "gone" or "more" Copies more words Chats – a mixture of words and babble	Points to some pictures in a book
Names 1-2 pictures in a book May join 2 words (daddy car, mummy go) Vocabulary increases	Understands many more words and instructions
Using short phrases "whassat" "there it is" "in there" Says own name	Can follow two commands "get my bag – it's in the hall"
Using some verbs as well as names "wash dolly" May combine 3 words	Copies his mother in his play (Puts doll in crib, etc.)
Says "me" or "mine"	Will listen to short stories
Beginning to tell you what he has done	Joins in short songs or rhymes

"I'm nearly two, there's lots I can do . . ."

Jumping and climbing

Your toddler is probably walking around steadily and speedily by now and can find his own way around his home and yard. He may want to find out what happens if he climbs on a chair, jumps off the bottom stair, turns that door handle, kicks or throws a ball, or trundles his sit-on toy down that slope. As he can move his body and limbs more freely and has better balance, by the age of two he will have added trotting or running, jumping and climbing to the many actions he can perform. His confidence will grow if you give him the opportunity to try out these new skills in safe ways. Watch him go up and come down the stairs and see how quickly his skill and confidence in moving build up. He may start by crawling up on his hands and scrambling down on his tummy, then progress to walking up and down one step at a time holding on. By the age of two he may be going up and down as you do.

Your toddler may now want to walk or take a favorite push-along toy with him when you go out. He'll trot along happily, stopping to look at every tree, gate or parked car on the way, so these trips can take quite a time! Take the stroller with you if you can, or you'll end up having to carry him and his toy as well.

Experimenting

Watch how he plays with smaller toys and you'll see that he wants to try out new things. He now has some idea of what he is trying to achieve. He may empty out a box full of small objects and fill it up again, sorting out and putting the objects back in order, using some pattern he has devised himself. He may also enjoy trying out some new tricks with familiar toys. Rolling toy cars down a gentle slope may keep him occupied for ages. Soon he'll be ready to move his cars in and out of a toy garage or line them up on a simple track. He'll also enjoy using his toys to copy some simple actions that he has seen happen. He may give his teddy bears a cup of pretend tea, for example, or put them to bed. These games will lead on to more complicated play later.

Using his hands

He can use his hands more skillfully now and activities which began only a few months ago have become a part of everyday play. Scribbles with a pencil show that he can make deliberate circular strokes and then change to make straight lines, the first steps in learning to draw. He can build taller towers with his blocks or line them up to make a low wall. Unscrewing tops of plastic jars may fascinate him and there are various toys which let him practice this and other actions where he has to use two hands together. Turning, twisting, pushing and pulling are all easy actions for his hands by this age.

He'll love sorting things out and matching them up. Although he is able to put objects of the same shape together, he may

Climbing is fun but always stay close when she's on equipment like this.

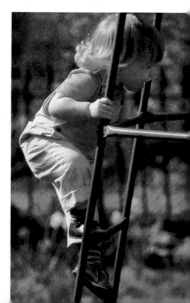

prefer to sort things out into lines or make his own patterns, and may get very frustrated if one of these objects is moved or sorted in a different way. By the age of two, and with only a little help from you, he will probably be able to match most of the shapes to the right holes in a simple sorting box and complete a board jigsaw with five or six pieces.

Looking after himself

Because he can understand so much more and can tell you things, as well as move efficiently and control his limbs, he can now take a greater part in looking after himself. Knowing the names of different parts of his body means he can "wash his face" or "take his socks off" when asked to do so. He may point to or even ask for things he wants to eat. If you offer him something he dislikes he can very definitely tell you he doesn't want it. He shows that he can choose just as adults do and that he can express that choice.

Toilet training. At this age some toddlers are ready to begin toilet training, though many will not be ready until they are two or over. Like any other skill, being able to control his bladder and bowel and make proper use of the toilet require a number of capabilities all working together. His muscles have to be sufficiently developed

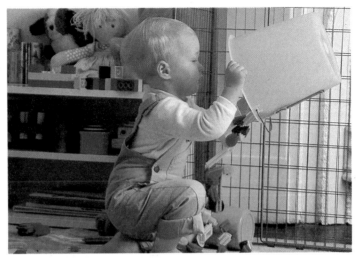

She'll enjoy getting toys out to play with – and might even help with putting them away.

to work when he tells them to, and he needs to remember and understand the sensation of being full in order to be able to tell you when he is ready to use the potty. Look for the signs that tell you he's ready to use the potty. He may not be able to use words, but his wriggles and strains suggest his awareness is developing. At first these signs may occur only after he has wet or dirtied his diaper. Have the potty close at hand so you can get him to it quickly when he shows you he may need it. When

he sits on it, give him sensible praise and cuddles if he produces anything. Don't show disappointment to him if nothing happens. How long it will take your toddler to become reliable in his habits is unpredictable. You provide the opportunity to learn this new skill but he will be the one to set the pace. It won't help if he feels rushed, so don't expect too much of him.

Sometimes toddlers start to show fussy or difficult behavior at this age, interfering with daily routines which have gone smoothly before. Try not to let him see that this upsets you or he may try it again to see your reaction.

NOW I CAN TALK (around 18 months to 2½ years)

	babbling →	understanding →	talking →
Making sense of the world	Experimenting with new ideas by himself	Trying out pretend games, e.g. tea party	
Whole body control	Starting to climb, jump and run	Kicking and throwing a ball in right direction Confident on stairs, goes up and down	
Looking	Looks at pictures in a book Follows what's going on	He looks at the details in pictures (puzzles and books) He follows actions from start to end	
Using his hands	He can build small towers with blocks Draw circles and straight lines	He can complete a simple shape, or a 5/6 piece inset puzzle Unscrews tops	
Listening and understanding	He can pick out certain toys when they are named He knows some parts of his body (hair, nose, feet)	He listens to short stories and can carry out simple instructions	
Communicating	Using single clear words amongst lots of chatter He wants to "tell" you about things	He may be using verbs as well as names Beginning to join words together	
Looking after himself	By himself he can sit at table, open doors Takes off hat, boots and arms out of coats	Starts to wash himself, and carry out simple dressing May be using potty Asks for what he wants when he has a choice	

The toddler's day

Your child will probably now be wanting a greater say in how he spends his day. Many 18-month-old toddlers will tell you in one way or another what they like to eat, to wear and play with. They may even be more adamant about what they don't like! It's at this age that your toddler gradually learns who's in charge and that this may vary depending on where he is and what's going on. He is learning too that sometimes he can have what he wants and sometimes he can't. He may love to run around barefoot, but if it's raining and he wants to go out then he must learn that he needs to put his shoes or boots on. He is beginning to be aware that there are rules about what is expected of him at different times.

Trying out all sorts of new games and activities is fun for your toddler, and the messier or noisier the game the more enjoyment it seems to give him! It can be very exasperating to find he has got out all his water pourers and has started to use them in that bucket of water you had left in the garden. He's bound to present himself soaked just as you were planning to go out for a visit. Planning your day is as important as ever, not so much in organizing his play for him, but

getting essential tasks done without too many upsets. If you are in a hurry to go out then it's unfair to let him get started on a game that takes a long time to set up or clear up. Put these toys out of sight to avoid disappointment.

Your willful toddler

No matter how well you plan things, there will inevitably be some disagreements over things he wants to do which are not allowed. Too many rules at any one time will confuse him and make life trying for both of you. Obviously it is important to keep strictly to the rules about his safety. Other rules need not be so strictly kept. He may be able to wander around eating a cookie if you have friends visiting and you can keep an eye on him, while at other times you may want him to sit at the table for his snack.

Giving him a long talking to about why he should not play with your pincushion or touch a hot oven door will mean little to him at this age. The tone of your voice alone tells him what you do not want him to do. A short warning such as "be careful" may caution him, or help him remember that things can hurt him. You could call your electrical outlets "Mr. Shocker" or your oven "Mr. Hot." Soon he may be warning himself: "Mr. Hot burns."

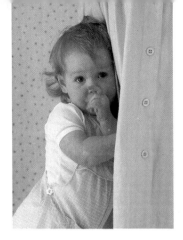

However willful and independent she may seem at times she still needs you there for comfort and security.

This age may be one of extremes for you and your child. One minute he's a happy and contented toddler whose company is a joy. The next he's angry or disappointed and you've no idea why. It's all part of coming to terms with his new independence. His increased abilities are themselves too much for him to cope with at times. Often he knows what he wants to do but the toys just won't go the right way or he is interrupted in a game before he can finish it. Try to understand his frustrations. Soon he will be able to explain better what is upsetting him. At the end of the day, remember the fun you've had together and the upsets will fall into perspective.

Toys and playthings

Despite the great changes in your child's development during his second year, many of the toys he already has will continue to be treasured possessions, though he may need you to show and encourage him to find new ways of playing with them. Teddy can be fitted with a baby hat or old sweater as well as being cuddled; blocks can be used for building a house for his playmen. Since he will want to try things out for himself as well, you will do best playing alongside him, making occasional suggestions.

Let's pretend

Some new puzzles, games or miniature household items may help him play and encourage him to chat away to himself or to his friends. When he speaks or tries to communicate using words or gestures, you become aware of how he is changing. He may pretend to be you, carrying out everyday routines with his toys, giving a doll a bath or talking on the telephone. The first signs that his play is becoming more imaginative is that he wants to give his teddy bear a drink, or use his wooden toy with wheels as a bus and then a truck. Watch him and you'll see that he is reliving events he has observed before. These are still early days in this type of play

and he will enjoy toys which are miniature versions of your things – a bag, a brush or a tool set. He is using his toys to mimic you and his friends.

Many of the best toys for this age are waiting in your cupboard – an old hat, bag, pair of shoes or worn-out shirt. Put on the hat or shoes yourself and pretend to be someone else; he'll soon get the idea. When you are buying something special for him, consider a stroller, tool kit, railway or set of play people or cars. Other toys that will continue to be popular at a later stage are a play house, kitchen set, ironing board, bath, or shop and cash register. Boys enjoy playing house, just as girls love train sets. Try to provide a wide variety of things to stimulate play. Play based on real life not only helps him to talk, but also to do things for himself and

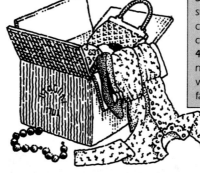

Toys to buy

1. Peg or play people, especially if in vehicles
2. Construction toys. Blocks that fit or screw together. Vehicles which hook together
3. Miniature household or everyday objects: a broom and pan, ironing board, tea set, cars and garages, simple train set
4. Puzzles and shape sorters. Choose one with about 6 to 8 pieces
5. Sand, shovels, buckets and pourers. A large container to hold the sand.

Toys you can make

1. A puppet. Use a wooden spoon and decorate it with a drawn face, with wool for hair, a paper skirt
2. Dressing up box. Hats, shoes, bags, cloaks are particularly popular at this age
3. Collection of bits and pieces for sticking and sorting. Empty cardboard boxes can be ships, cars or stoves.
4. Make his own corner. All you need is a blanket over a table, with a cushion and some favorite toys inside.

learn new skills. He may learn to undo the buttons on his teddy bear's shirt or pull a shoe lace undone.

Playing with other children

At this stage other children are as important for play as toys, especially if your child is the first or only child. Play with others will help him learn new things, encourage him to talk and later to share and take turns. It is never easy at first and you may feel that your outings to friends' houses become battlegrounds. But it is worth persevering. The day will come when he will actually enjoy letting a friend have a go on his bike! This social play begins with his play with you. You can lift him, copy him, race with him, sing rhymes, or play games with him. If you join in his play with other children he can see how you share, chat, enjoy the company of others and introduce new games. Two children together can learn to ride on a seesaw, play tug-of-war or ball games. Remember, it's a big step from playing alongside another child to joining in a game and sharing a toy with them.

Making his toys work

His growing capabilities mean that he can enjoy puzzles or toys which help him learn how to solve problems, sort out similar shapes or pictures, or find out how new things work. He'll come to grips with toy record players, toys with knobs which turn and parts to pull, tool benches with hammers, screwdrivers and screws. He'll use his stacking beakers or your plastic boxes to find out how they fit inside one another, or how high he can build them. He may try to match all the green or red ones. He is beginning to put new parts of his building sets together. All the time he is trying out ideas to see if they work. Shape puzzles and sorting boxes are also popular.

Toys that help your child to use her imagination will be very popular now. She loves copying what you do and will create pretend situations that copy her real life. A tea party is fun and she'll chat away to herself.

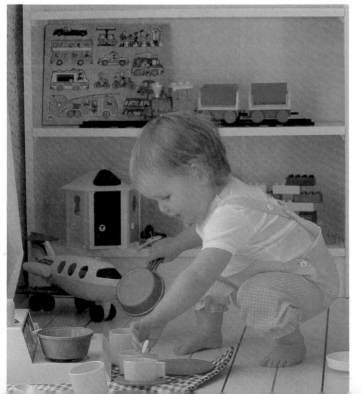

Games toddlers enjoy

Watch your toddler play and you'll see how busy he is trying out new games for himself. He may still want to be near you, but won't want you to do so many things for him or interrupt his game.

Having fun together

Making some comments on what he is doing, or showing him a new game when he is tired of his own, will be more helpful to him and stretch his concentration. For example, if he has been rolling some empty cardboard tubes around the floor, and looks bored, pick one up and put one of his small bricks down it. He'll then want to discover for himself which of his toys will fit and roll out on to the floor. If he is busily engrossed in a game he may take little notice of you or get angry if you take something he needs. Be careful about deciding when to join in. Sometimes he may need you to help in practical ways. He may be too small to carry a big box over to the table, so you are called upon to help out; but don't go too far and spoil his fun by opening up the box. He can do that for himself. You'll be asked to step in for games that need two players. Rolling a ball or hide-and-seek cannot easily be played without a partner to enter into the

Safety

The 18-24-month-old appears to be capable of so much it is easy to overestimate his understanding of situations.

- He will probably not realize what words such as "hot," "sharp," "high" really mean yet, and if he does he may easily forget when he is busy playing. Stoves, fires, knives, scissors, boxes of pins, hot water faucets, unsteady tables or walls are just some of the things he may need protection from. Remember he may be able to climb now so he can reach up to shelves and cupboards that were too high for him before.

- He may be quite confident on the stairs now but a guard might still be necessary if he cannot be watched or if he is in someone else's house and the stairs are not familiar to him. He may wake at night and a stairgate may stop him falling if he can get out of bed.

- He may not realize his own strength when playing with other children. He may throw something, push or hit another child and not be aware of the outcome. He may get careless if he gets over-excited; for example, if he's running to see something special he may trip or run into something. You can't leave toddlers unsupervised for long.

- Learning to hold hands near roads is now especially important.

- At the park, watch for him climbing up the big slide or gym before he is ready. You may need to follow up behind. Be careful he does not run too close to moving swings and get hit.

- Make sure he uses wheeled toys appropriately. If trodden on or climbed on they will slip away from under him and he will fall off.

- Remember he can get to most places now and can turn door handles or push locks across. He may shut himself in a room and become frightened or open the front door and run out on to a busy road.

fun and share the game.

He will enjoy games with different material – playdough, sand and water. Even when it is too cold to play outside, bath time is an opportunity for water games.

Out and about

Going out is always an adventure in your toddler's life and suggests new ideas for games to play. The park may always look the same to you but he'll see something different every time. Talking about these things at the time and pointing out similar things in his books later on at home make the outing more memorable. When another child comes to play, plan a game that they can both play on their own, but alongside each other, to help avoid battles over both wanting the same toy. A box of crayons and paper may keep the two occupied for quite a while. Your toddler's favorite toy may have to be put away on these visits as this is something he will find it impossible to share. At a toddler group you can watch him learning how to play games with other children. He'll probably choose to stay near one or two particular friends. They may offer each other toys or enjoy a noisy run-around game, all shouting the same noise.

Books and quiet games

There will still be times in your busy toddler's day when he will want to sit with you, playing quieter games. Get out his picture books and tell him some of the names of pictures or see if he can point to the picture of the "boy in

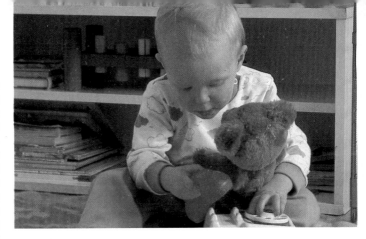

Talking on the telephone is fun – and teddy wants to have a word too!

the hat" or the "red ball." Many happy minutes can be spent like this, and it's a good way to spend time waiting at the doctor's or on a journey.

Making up a story or collecting items for a scrapbook can make quiet games last longer and help him feel more involved.

Simple counting games, such as saying the rhyme "1-2-3-4-5, Once-I-caught-a-fish-alive" while touching each of his fingers in turn, may encourage him to try and repeat the words. Showing your pleasure at his attempts to repeat words will make him want to try again. He may join in parts of other rhymes but probably cannot manage all the words yet.

Pretend games

Playing games where his dolls or teddy bears "talk" to each other may tempt him to chatter away. Perhaps you could "work" one

dolly and he another, and have a simple tea party. Using puppets is another version of this and he will like them just as much if they are made at home from a wooden spoon with a face drawn on it. He may enjoy dressing up from that collection of old clothes, bags and shoes which you could put together. Ask him questions about his costume. "Have you got your hat on?" "Are you daddy going to work?" "Is it raining outside?"

It is from everyday activities and playtimes that ideas for the best games arise, the ones that will hold his interest most strongly. In these imaginary situations he can practice the skills he needs in real life and increase his confidence at tackling new tasks.

Some songs and rhymes

1 2 3 4 5

One, two, three, four, five,
Once I caught a fish alive,
Six, seven, eight, nine, ten,
Then I let it go again.
Why did you let it go?
Because it bit my finger so.
Which finger did it bite?
This little finger on the right.

The itsy bitsy spider

The itsy bitsy spider
Climbed up the water spout;
Down came the rain
And washed the spider out:
Out came the sun
And dried up all the rain;
And the itsy bitsy spider
Climbed up the spout again.

Ride-a-cock-horse

Ride-a-cock-horse to Banbury Cross,
To see a fine lady upon a white horse;
With rings on her fingers and bells on her toes,
She shall have music wherever she goes.

Two little dicky birds

Two little dicky birds
Sitting on a wall,
One named Peter
The other named Paul
Fly away Peter!
Fly away Paul!
Come back Peter!
Come back Paul!

Round and round the garden

Round and round the garden
Like a teddy bear
One step, two step,
And tickle you under there!

Pat-a-cake

Pat-a-cake, pat-a-cake, baker's man,
Bake me a cake as fast as you can;
Pat it and prick it, and mark it with B
And toss it in the oven for baby and me.

Rub-a-dub-dub

Rub-a-dub-dub,
Three men in a tub,
And who do you think they be?
The butcher, the baker,
The candlestick-maker,
Turn 'em out, knaves all three!

This little piggy

This little piggy went to market,
This little piggy stayed home,
This little piggy had roast beef,
And this little piggy had none,
And this little piggy cried Wee, wee, wee, wee
All the way home.

Ring-around-the-rosy

Ring-around-the-rosy,
A pocket full of posies,
Ashes, ashes
We all fall down.

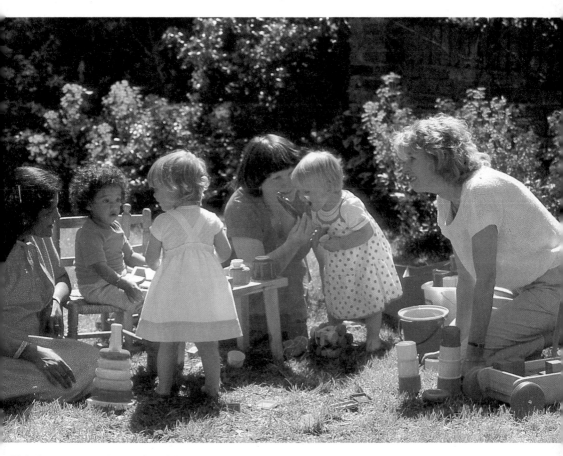

This is the way the ladies ride

This is the way the ladies ride,
Tri, tre, tre, tree,
Tri, tre, tre, tree;
This is the way the ladies ride,
Tri, tre, tre, tre, tri-tre-tre-tree!

This is the way the gentlemen ride
Gallop-a-trot,
Gallop-a-trot,
This is the way the gentlemen ride,
Gallop-a-gallop-a-trot!

This is the way the farmers ride,
Hobbledy-hoy,
Hobbledy-hoy,
This is the way the farmers ride,
Hobbledy, hobbledy-hoy!

63

Index

ACKNOWLEDGMENTS

Photography by Sandra Lousada, assisted by Daphne Wright and Susanna Price. The publishers would like to thank Young World, Early Learning Centre, Harrods, Galt Toys, Patrick's for the loan of toys.
Illustrations by Elsa Willson.